THE
CAGED
GIANT

From Victim through Survivor to Thriver

MANYI EBOT

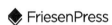

Suite 300 - 990 Fort St
Victoria, BC, V8V 3K2
Canada

www.friesenpress.com

ISBN
978-1-5255-3545-1 (Hardcover)
978-1-5255-3546-8 (Paperback)
978-1-5255-3547-5 (eBook)

1. SELF-HELP, ABUSE

Distributed to the trade by The Ingram Book Company

DEDICATION

To all trauma victims, survivors and thrivers out there. Use your voice; live your dreams!

Your investment in this book will provide psychosocial assistance like formal education, skills development, and housing to trauma survivors.

Grateful for you!

INTRODUCTION

A while ago, my daughter who was four years old at the time asked a question, which awakened my core. Her tender fingers tapped my feet then she looked up to me searchingly and said, "Mom, when you were a kid, what did you want to be when you grow up?"

I looked at her, smiled and continued my chores. Possibly assuming I did not understand her question, she went on to ask again with an explanation. "Mom, when you were a child what did you want to be when you grew up? Did you want to be a teacher, a doctor, or a police officer? This time I laughed and said, "Sweetheart, I am already grown up."

My persistent little girl didn't give up on her questions but this experience was an awakening moment in my life. Although my response showed that we sometimes settle for where we are because of age and circumstances leaving so much potential untapped, this discussion also provoked a thought which lingered longer than expected.

When children are asked questions like this in their early childhood some will talk about careers they want to get into but what others really hope for is just to be in a safe environment. What they want is to get away from that abusive relative, neighbor or to grow up and move away from the neglect and/or loss.

In their adulthood, they may fulfill their dream but those earlier circumstances leave other repercussions. Many are left with the loss of self, memory and/or future aspirations in their post-traumatic lives.

The purpose of this book is to explore the core concerns and provide a valuable resource on the pathway of recovery. The victimization of trauma may have made you believe you are who you are not. It is imperative to get another view in your reassessment for the recollection of the self, history and your destiny. Hopefully, this will be a valuable tool in your toolbox to connect with you at the stage you are in – be it a victim or survivor – and support you to thrive.

The aim is to walk with you as you create the best version of yourself. It is easy to get stuck in whom you were or didn't have the chance to be; to get caught up in what you certainly didn't deserve. However, a shift can be made in the direction you desire and deserve. Welcome on board with us to find out how to make that shift.

No matter what you have been through, you are not alone.

No matter what you have been through, you are not alone. That is why the book starts with the lived experience of Kiki and every chapter has a segment called Journey with Kiki. The content might be triggering to anyone with similar experiences, but it is important to explore this in depth insight into trauma.

As we journey with Kiki, we get the chance to see how the topic of discussion in that chapter is applied to a person's experience. This provides a guide on how you can apply the write-up to your situation.

No matter the state you are in at the moment, I believe you have the power, abilities, and control to recreate your life. You can be in the driver's seat of your life and steer it in the direction of your choice. Your life is too valuable to be left in the hands of chance and other people.

This truth inspired most chapters to end with questions of reflection. It is my prayer that you will find the answers to these questions within you, get out of the cage and explore all the potential you are graciously endowed with.

PROLOGUE

Excitedly, the young lady rushed through the flourishing bushes that had grown on the path to the house her husband inherited from his grandfather as the first grandson. Right now, the state of the house didn't matter much to her as it had in the few years they had lived in it, though she always sighed saying, "It is much better than paying rent, which we probably would never have been able to afford for a decent property."

She tried to bring her mind back to the reality of what had just happened. It all seems like a dream, one she hopes she never wakes up from.

Just like her parents, Kiki and her siblings grew up in a small city of less than two hundred thousand people. Her parents' education and careers placed her family in a higher standard of living compared to more than three-quarters of the population in her city. This made her the envy of her peers. Little did they know that all that glitters is not always gold. No one could imagine the pain in her heart caused by the dangerous forces in the world.

Part of it could be imagined through the tragedy that took her parents' lives, the day they died on the spot at a ghastly car accident. The devastation from the loss plunged the once vibrant princess into solitude, and deeper despair to add to the low self-esteem she was already facing from experiences she dared not recount.

All this she expected to change when she met a young college graduate with whom she fell in love. Barely six months later, they decided
to get married against the advice of both families who believed the
couple needed more time to get to know each other. This advice fell on
deaf ears as the couple stood on the point that they know each other
better than those who got married simply because their families paired
them together. On Kiki's path, she was more excited to meet someone
who in her opinion would fill in the gap of the loss she felt after the
departure of her parents from this world.

Two years into the marriage, the couple realized that they had
underestimated the challenge of being united without a stable source of
income. At this time, she had just obtained her bachelor's degree thanks
to the benevolence of her extended family members but now the tables
had been turned to her as the caregiver of her three teenage siblings
who relied on their sole source of income – her husband's irregular
meager salary – for their basic needs.

Her gratitude for the joy she feels at the moment goes back to the day
she met a former classmate. After exchanging pleasantries, this friend
told her about a number of scholarship positions available to further
her studies abroad if she is selected. Her friend gave her the online
link, telling her she has applied and praying she will be selected. In the
days that unfolded after the meeting, Kiki flooded the schools with
applications with the hope to fill in at least one position in any school
irrespective of the country.

For several months, she checked her email at least twenty times a day
in expectancy of an acceptance letter. She had been dreaming of having
a better life anywhere else except in her country of birth. She hoped
for a silver lining to peek through her cloud of loss, pain, despair, and
anguish, which had almost completely wiped away her beautiful early
memories of the treasures she once possessed.

Unexpectedly, the moment she had been waiting for came through
at a time she had lost hope and checked her emails occasionally rather

than out of anticipation. She could hardly breathe in anxiety as she opened the acceptance letter to study at a prestigious university in one of her enviable countries in the world. The light became brighter as she read further to discover that her scholarship covered her tuition for the entire two years of studies.

Unsure of how she would get there, one thing she was sure of is that this is the glimmer of hope she had been searching for most of her adult life. Her celebration couldn't go uninterrupted as worry set in on how to raise the money for her flight and secondly, will her husband of five years accompany her abroad? She fought the worry by telling herself that notwithstanding, their lives are going to get better.

It did seem to get better when after lots of inquiries, they came to the knowledge that he could accompany her on a spousal work permit.

Bilah her husband, a graduate with a BSc in Biochemistry worked as a laboratory technician in a private clinic in their city of residence. Due to the inability of a majority of their clients to pay their bills, Bilah often goes for months without being paid the few thousands he expects to receive monthly. As such, the family spends the evening and Saturdays working on the piece of the land he inherited from his deceased father.

This land, which has been the main supply of their food is their last resort to raise funds for their travel. Without hesitation, they began the search for a buyer to purchase their means of survival in order to raise the money for the processing of their visas and purchase of their flight tickets.

Kiki didn't have a lot of people to turn to in her moment of need. Her parents' families have been fighting over the properties left behind with little consideration of the children of the deceased.

After paying her way through the university, they had left her to fend for her younger siblings though she had not been able to secure a job upon graduation.

The proceeds from the land were barely enough to cover their expenses as they didn't get as much as they had anticipated due to the urgency of selling the land. However, nothing could stop them from making the journey.

After all the hustle, the eve of their departure finally arrived. Surrounded by friends and family members who came to wish them goodbye, Kiki was alone in her thoughts; drowned in her daydreaming of the glamorous life she saw awaiting her in her future environment.

She could see Bilah working at a sophisticated laboratory in an extremely large hospital making lots and lots of money such that they will be able to own a modern luxurious mansion both home and abroad, drive the latest cars and she will finally find a solution to their sex problem, the reason she believes explains why she has not been able to get pregnant after five years in marriage. After all, she expects the medical practitioners there to know everything.

She could hardly imagine the joy of holding children from her womb. Now she sees a brighter future opening up for them; a future where her children will get the best education without their parents having sleepless nights on how to pay for it. There was also a possibility for her to buy those beautiful toys she has been admiring on the Internet, wishing she had kids who could play with them though sighing that she may never be able to afford it even if she had children of her own.

Her daydreaming paused as she had to bid her guests farewell, apologizing that they didn't have enough money to rent a bus so all their loved ones could accompany them to the airport. Some people expressed their dismay for not being able to accompany them so they can see the airport for the first time in their lives. Others were just very happy that Kiki and Bilah were going to greener pastures to breathe fresh air.

She barely slept that night but found herself continuing her dream of their life abroad during the few hours she dozed off intermittently.

After two full years in her dreamland, it dawned on her that life was nothing compared to what she had dreamed about. Things she had never imagined found their way into her reality. What astonished her most was the question she had to answer every single day of her life – where are you from? Which was often followed by, what is your first language?

Her first words had been in English. That is the only language she has ever spoken. Yet because of her accent, which she didn't know she had until this stage in her life, this question often caused her to zoom into the childhood she dreaded in order to answer a question she didn't think necessary.

As though that was not enough of a problem for her, for the first time in her life, she had gone for days without food, though without voluntarily fasting. This was extremely important so she could squeeze out whatever dollars could drip from her student job paycheck after meeting their expenses so she could send some money to her siblings back home for their education.

Bilah had not been able to get a job in his field as he often received the response that he didn't have any work experience in his country of residence, to qualify for him for at least one of the hundreds of job interviews he had been to.

Following the advice of a friend and the tension in their marriage caused by the financial struggle, he decided to accept a job as a warehouse attendant in a production company. Though it was not his ideal job, at least it gave him reasons to reinstate his pride as a responsible African man who takes care of his family. That may have been sufficient if it was the only reason for his growing pride but they just found out that they will be having a baby in eight months.

At last, his family and friends will now know that he is indeed a man. The murmurs, rumors, advice and insults of their infertility will get weaker as Kiki's tummy protrudes out daily. They were indeed grateful that what had seemed impossible for seven years had become possible today, though they both knew there was more to their childlessness than what the naysayers discerned.

Their gratitude list just got longer with Kiki at the verge of completing her studies. Her life had been a marathon for the past two years: studying, working, visiting doctors and her school counselor to make all this success a reality. Nevertheless, she had mapped out the next phase of her life without sharing her plans with her husband.

On April 12, her twin girls saw the world for the first time shortly after her graduation ceremony. It had been a very difficult pregnancy so the joy was overflowing to see an end of the pregnancy while welcoming her bundles of joy. This spring hope sparked more visions from Kiki who was determined to spend every single day glued to her children for the first months of their life and get a job with her freshly achieved master's degree as soon as she can.

While they transitioned into parenthood, it was also a time to make a change in their residency status. Though both changes didn't come easy, the change into motherhood was unbearable for Kiki who had little support from her husband, primarily due to his work at night and sleeping all day to refresh before going for another night shift.

She desperately missed her close-knit family and community. She never thought raising kids in a foreign country was so much different from the way she had seen kids raised in her country of origin, a place where it truly took a community to raise a child. Now she doubted the statement she always heard growing up, "The most difficult part of motherhood is being pregnant; once the baby is born, the work is done."

Of course, that could be true in the part of the world where she was born. A place where a mother could go for hours without seeing her baby yet she is at peace because she is certain her baby will be handed to her safely by one of the numerous volunteer caregivers on standby, all waiting for a turn to look after the baby.

Less than a week after the birth of the twins, the joy they brought along was slowly giving way to a deep feeling of sadness. It all started with Kiki silently shedding tears that her parents didn't live to see her babies. She yearned for the support she could have gotten from her mother. As if being sad about the lack of family support was not enough for her deal with, she constantly found herself in a low mood every time her breast could not come up with enough milk to feed her babies; a mood that moved from occasionally to almost a constant sensation.

Kiki had strongly decided to exclusively breastfeed her babies, as she had fantasized and also what she had learned in her culture and tradition. The struggle to produce more milk continued as did her mood, sinking her deeper into despair. For the sake of her children's survival, she finally gave in to supplement their feeding. However, she felt anxious each time she picked up a prepared bottle of formula to feed her babies.

This anxiety opened up a wound of self-condemnation, one she had fought so hard to heal but was still in the process of patching. A feeling which only triggered memories of worthlessness, the same way she had felt in her childhood when her father repeatedly raped her on several occasions.

It was a time in her life she had fought so hard never to remember. A time when her yet to recover self-esteem had been shattered after she summed up the courage to tell her mother about the sexual assault, only for her mother to turn around and accuse her of walking around the house half naked with the aim of seducing her husband.

It was a time when her parents had lavished her with glamorous gifts to buy her silence in order to save the family name from shame and disgrace without much consideration given to her own life.

It was a time she wished had washed away with the past or gone with her parents from the earth yet it has always shown up in her present. She had almost lost her marriage because she couldn't bear her husband touching her. It was the reason she had been unable to conceive within the few years of marriage.

Although she is not sure if her hatred for her husband's touch was a result of her father's action or the female genital mutilation she had gone through months before the initial sexual abuse.

Today, she attributes her victory to her school counselor with whom she spoke occasionally. The sweet lady who went outside her job description to help her build romance in her marriage.

That first year of being a mother, which she had thought was going to be fun-filled turned out to be tears-filled. Like in her childhood, she found herself once again taking the blame and accepting the guilt for the babies' cries, their challenge with feeding and the reason for them appearing hurt.

Bilah, on the other hand, was too busy to notice his wife's pain and struggle while she was too scared to talk about her experiences with anyone. If there is one thing she feared most, it was being judged and labeled.

After weeks of thinking about a solution, she resolved to get a job, put her children in childcare, believing that going out daily and having something to look forward to besides her children will help boost her mood. Besides, she desperately needs the income to give her immediate and extended family a better standard of living.

Little did she know that this new plan was going to be the onset of trouble in her home. Breathlessly, she explained her plan to her husband in between his wake-up time and time to go to work. Without much consideration, Bilah said a firm NO, adding that Kiki should never consider working for he has decided that she will stay home and raise their children.

Every effort to convince him to change his mind turned fruitless. The resistance from her husband escalated into other family conflicts, which always ended in verbal and domestic violence. With her hopes of getting out of the house to face the day being dashed, she resolved to stay in the house all day and hide from the world.

Alone, she carried the weight of the childhood trauma, domestic abuse and her deteriorating mental health and marriage. This weight pressed on every reason she had to take care of herself.

The once neat Kiki who had a special touch at turning every messy place into a spotless palace and making every piece of clothing an object of fashion admiration, started going for weeks without a shower or change of clothes.

Bilah, who now spent days out before returning home, showed no interest in her. The few words he ever offered were to nag her for her neglect of self-care, which he interpreted as laziness, dirtiness, negligence and incompetence as a mother and wife. He often added she is not the first person to bear children so she should pull herself together.

Kiki's fear about opening up concerning her situation grew stronger for she concluded that everyone will treat her just like her husband. From knowledge obtained, she could perceive that she needed to get help but couldn't face asking anyone for it. She dreaded that the outcome might lead to her greatest nightmare.

Years went by, taking away more of her happiness with it while her daily living moved from bad to worse. The day finally came when her fake smiles could no longer come into existence as she broke out in tears to a "mommy acquaintance" who seemed to show her genuine concern each time she dropped off and picked up her kids from school.

Her "miracle friend" advised her to seek help for the sake of her life and to be present to watch her children grow up. After a lot of resistance, she finally gave in to her concerned friend, who introduced her to a safe community. A community that did not see her as a broken woman that needed fixing but a woman with lots of strengths and potential to produce the best version of herself with the right support – one they were willing to offer.

CHAPTER 1:
THE WIRING

"When you find yourself in a new situation, a new circumstance, a new life experience, everything that requires healing is going to rush to the surface."
—*Iyanla Vanzant*

Kiki's story in the opening pages of this book could be something you have never heard or imagined so you are wondering; could this be a true story or a fantasy? Well, it is okay if you are not familiar with such details but sadly, millions of people can relate to that story either as survivors of one or more slices of her life, the experiences of their loved ones or as trauma-informed practitioners.

I am always asked the question – what is trauma?

When I started this conversation about trauma – mostly with folks from third world countries, who are academically educated and have had a level of exposure – to know if stories like Kiki's or mine was unique or are we not just talking about it, what struck me is that I am always asked the question – what is trauma?

Up until that point, I had taken for granted that everyone knows about it. It then became evident that trauma is not something given enough attention as it should yet it is a busy road with many travelers. A vast majority use the word without giving much thought to it, others have experienced it without having a name for it. It is particularly easy to know it because of the many circumstances where it originates:

- Abuse in childhood; emotional, physical or sexual
- Accidents: Automobile, physical activity
- Abandonment
- Being robbed or witnessing violent crime
- Betrayal and inability to stand up for yourself
- Bullying and defamation of character
- Cultural displacement including voluntarily moving to the diaspora
- Depression including post-partum depression
- Domestic violence
- Terrorism, war and displacement.
- Natural disasters
- Losing a loved one through death, separation or divorce
- Substance use and addiction
- Traditional practices such as female genital mutilation
- Loss of a stable source of income
- Poverty
- Medical procedures and illnesses

Despite the length of this list drawn from personal experience and the experiences of those who kindly shared their stories, it is not exhaustive. The diversity in tracing the cause of trauma makes it more complex to come up with a definition for it. This is because within every story is embedded a definition.

However, the underlying denominator is that it is any undesirable life event which occurs in a state of helplessness and obstructs the likelihood to recognize or maximize abilities and skills. These events may have happened to almost everyone at one point or another in life but the distinguishing factor is that we all respond to them differently at different times.

This is okay because there are no two people with the same DNA. I am not a scientist so I don't know much about DNA except one thing for sure, which is that it is unique for each person, so we can't all have the same coping mechanisms.

The results from these events could go unnoticed but in most cases it leads to;

- Anger
- Avoidance behaviors
- Anxiety
- Always expecting the worst
- Bouts of flashback and nightmares
- Dependency
- Despair
- Fear
- Feelings of unworthiness
- Impaired decision making
- Numbness
- Sensitive to noise or touch
- Stress
- Unexplainable physical pain

If a person has a cut on their arm, we consider that cut recovered when the impaired skin becomes operational, the excruciating pain, which could not be ignored, is no longer there and in some cases, the scars have been erased. But how can we point out the recovery of a person who was raped several years ago, was physically and verbally maltreated by their abusers, moved on to live in isolation and is in a constant state of sadness?

This is not something you can see like physical scars, which are no longer present. It is not a conclusion you can jump into based on your observation without looking at it from the person's perspective. It is not something you can treat without genuinely accepting the role of a supporter irrespective of your own point of view. In other words, it is not a one size fit all but a person-to-person approach.

So, what is trauma? Interestingly, the word trauma is derived from a Greek word, which means wound. Just like physical wounds, trauma is a term used to describe our internal wounds. However, while almost everyone will agree that a person with a physical wound can recover, the same is not true for a survivor of the unseen wound because many have a contrary opinion.

FACTS ABOUT WOUNDS

1. **Broken Barrier**

A cut occurs when there is a tearing on the surface of the skin, which is a barrier meant to protect the tissues and organs beneath it. This implies that the safeguard has been broken exposing a delicate organ to a limited defense to external forces.

Reflection
- The skin is just a surface concealing the body parts that lie within, if an external object passes through it and harms what it conceals, will you expect the bearer to respond like nothing ever happened?
- Does a broken skin, which is a broken barrier mean a broken person?

2. **Depth and Size**

Some cuts on the skin are seen only on the surface. If some kind of device is used to look into the body, it will be seen that the wound did not go beyond the skin. Others will reveal through the monitoring device that the wound has damaged the dermis, the underlying muscles, fat and in some cases the damage goes as far as the bones.

Also, the external wound doesn't always reveal its depth, neither does it expose the concreteness of the harm caused. Some wounds cover a little portion on the surface of the skin while others are generous in their use of the skin. Wounds come in different sizes and depths.

Reflection
- How deep is your wound? Is it shallow and can only be seen on the surface or deep down within, more than anyone can imagine?

3. External Forces

All wounds are caused by an external object. It could be an internal wound, a split of the organs in the body. However, one thing is certain, that wound was caused by another object which had contact with the injured.

Reflection
- Would it be justifiable for the injured to take full responsibility for the injury it is experiencing?

4. Attention Administered

After the division of the skin comes a process whereby the broken pieces have to repair and restore the strength and functionality of the damaged tissue. Based on the state of the dermis, the wound can be cured using basic first aid. If it is a more advanced damage, more intense medical attention will be required. The point here is that not all wounds require medical attention but all wounds deserve an observation.

Reflection
- Are you a parent, teacher, coach or a person in authority besides a medical practitioner? Have you ever administered a first aid procedure to someone who has been injured, even a procedure as simple as wiping off the bleeding and assured the person that everything is going to be okay?
- How did the injured respond to the treatment you offered?

5. Wound Infection

There are cases where a wound that was not properly treated gets infected and more complicated to treat. Perhaps the wound didn't receive proper hygiene after attention, was treated with a contaminated object or an incorrect treatment was administered. All these results in undesirable outcomes which could be a foul smell, liquid draining out of it or more pain than was originally present. It could also be evident visually that something is not right through the visible inflamed surrounding areas. Worse still, an infection can lead to a permanent or temporary challenge preventing the injured part from functioning to full potential.

Reflection
- Can the relationship between two parts be severed because the infection from one party caused a reaction from the injured? Could this influence the injured to involuntarily respond in ways that create an impediment between the two parties?
- Have you ever inexperienced a situation where you had a hindrance in using a part of you which was temporary or permanently infected? How did you respond to that experience?

> Ignoring the signs or symptoms won't make the wound go away.

6. Signs and Symptoms

Every ailment announces itself through signs and symptoms so wounds are no exceptions and just like any other, signs are detected by any observer while symptoms are only known to its bearer. In some cases, it is easy to miss this duo because they are so obvious that they are not taken as something which could be of serious concern or they have simply been there for too long. Ignoring the signs or symptoms won't make the wound go away.

Wounds show signs like bleeding and swelling depending on their kind and symptoms like pain which can best be expressed by the individual experiencing it. Don't take the pain for granted if the symptom is not on you.

Reflection
- Is it possible to tell how much pain a person is undergoing just by watching the individual?

7. Concurrent Ailment

There are some moments when there is a pain-filled bleeding wound you are trying to deal with but not able to fully focus on it as you should because at that same moment there is maybe a migraine or a fever whose symptoms are stronger though unrelated to the wound. As such, they are cohabitants of the same body.

Imaginably, it would have been a little bit easier to deal with one ailment at a time but unfortunately, that luxury doesn't always fall into place.

Reflection
- If concurrent ailments occur in the body, do they also exist in the mind, soul or whatever you choose as the residence of trauma?
- If yes, it is okay to provide help for one ailment without doing as little as glancing towards the direction of the other(s)?

8. Wound History

Is it just me or does this happen to everyone else? From personal experience with serious cuts and other times I accompanied a wounded person to a medical facility for treatment, the following questions are always asked:

- How long has this wound lasted?
- Have there been any changes since the onset of this wound?
- Have you had any wounds in the past?

Sometimes in the midst of the pain, these questions sound annoying, particularly when asked prior to offering any remedy. Out of pain coupled with curiosity, I had to demand why these questions have to be asked. The answer may give you the same shock it gave me.

It is important to know a person's history of the present and past wounds in order to provide the best treatment and security, get information about previous treatments used, longevity to heal and complications which may have arisen or perceived to arise and how to commence the present treatment.

Personal stories are characteristic of everyone. It is beneficial to release them as opposed to holding on to them in order to get the right treatment.

Reflection
- How can an understanding of your past play a role in the recovery of your present wounds?
- What effects can an incomplete, improper or wrong treatment of a past wound have in the prognosis of a present wound?

9. Wound Recovery

Specific types determine the different treatments and journey of recovery. I believe if all wounds are treated with the same method, some will heal faster than others while others will remain stagnant or get worse. I assume the goal of every person administering treatment is to heal the wound to the extent that it allows the injured part to return to normal function.

In some cases, the injured part needs to be sewed to bind the broken pieces, thereby picking up the shattered and move on in recovery. Avoiding the needle, in this case, won't help the wound heal. It could work in other injuries like scratches in some individuals where the skin could repair itself to normal functioning with little or no intervention.

The wound is just like any other wound, which can recover, but every recovery is unique.

Reflection
Examine this scenario.

A robber holding a gun walks into a bank with twenty people present. He points the gun from one direction to another demanding that everyone hands their wallet, purse, briefcase or whatever case that contains money. He turns to the tellers and demands them to turn in all the cash in the register.

Two minutes later, he spots law enforcement officers surrounding the place. Out of frustration and confusion, he begins shooting randomly. In the commotion, some people run in search of safety, fall and get injured from furniture, others suffer from gunshots but no lives are lost.

Finally, the robber is apprehended and calm is restored in the bank.

Do you think all twenty people will recount the same story in the exact same words?

- Will they all have the same kind of wounds?
- Will they all have the same journey of recovery from this external force, which has invaded what seemed to be the normal course of their day?

RECOVERY IS POSSIBLE

Trauma is a wound in the mind, which if not properly treated at the time of occurrence is always present to prevent a person from reaching their full potential.

Irrespective of the opinion you have when it comes to trauma recovery, I would like you to note one thing: Recovery is possible! If there is one statement you will take away from this book, it should be this: Recovery is possible!

If you are a perpetrator of the belief that recovery is impossible, there is no need to be frightened because I once shared your belief, especially dealing with the aftermath of my own traumatic experiences. The question is what caused the mindset change?

PSYCHOSOCIAL REHABILITATION

My contact with psychosocial rehabilitation was my first contact with the recovery paradigm. I totally understand if your reaction to the phrase above is "what is that?" That is the initial response I get most often when I mention it. So before you choose to skip this portion of the book thinking it might not be relevant to you, let's dive into the words of Corrigan et al., "…the broad set of practices that comprise psychiatric[psychosocial] rehabilitation are equally meaningful for the general population in dealing with the day-to-day problems that occur in everyone's lives" (2009, ix)

That said, what is psychosocial rehabilitation? "Psychosocial rehabilitation (also termed psychiatric rehabilitation or PSR) promotes personal recovery, successful community integration and satisfactory quality of life for persons who have a mental illness or mental health concern."[1]

What I find intriguing about this is that I have come across several beliefs, backgrounds, cultures, and traditions, which consider mental health concerns including trauma to be a death sentence. They have often been regarded as something that renders a person permanently incapable of ever having a thriving and meaningful life; whatever that means to you.

The contact with a paradigm that advocates **hope**, **recovery** and **empowerment** for all persons sets the ball rolling to rethinking personal philosophies that have set limitations on so many achievements.

A better understanding of this concept will require looking deeper into this trio:

Hope
Hope to me is the driving force to take that next step despite the current situation. It is the reason why when there is not enough convincing evidence that everything is going to be okay yet, goals, dreams and visions are extended from this present into the future even if the goal is just to wake up the next morning. Therefore, taking a stance in hope gives the assurance that despite the challenges there is a possibility that the best days are not in the past.

> Moving from the bottom of a ladder to the top is a process, and I consider every step from one level to the next to be a recovery ...

Recovery

This is a tricky one because it can frustrate hope depending on the dimension looked at. I like to look at it as a ladder. Moving from the bottom of a ladder to the top is a process, and I consider every step from one level to the next to be a recovery because at every step, an attribute necessary for a personally satisfying life which was lost or never present is (re)introduced or enhanced.

On the other hand, if recovery is only considered to take place when the person is at the top of the ladder, then the results of hope, which is worth celebrating along the journey, will be lost and perhaps many will give up on the way.

A measurement for recovery that has been personally inspirational is the PROM (Personal Recovery Outcome Measure) model designed by Dr. Skye Barbic, Associate Professor at the University of British Columbia[2].

This model comes with a questionnaire and a ruler. The participant is required to answer 30 questions, followed by indicating the score on the ruler after doing some mathematics. You may have figured out that math is surely not one of my passions, and you are right about that. Anyway, back to our PROM.

The sweet part about it is that you indicate your score after the math on a ruler. Based on your score, the participant or practitioner comes up with an assessment or goals to further improve the score.

This is my best part of PROM because no matter how often I measure my recovery, there is always room for improvement, which is an indicator to me that there is a better part of me worth looking forward to and it could mean the same for you unless you get the full score – in which case I would like to meet you! That leads to the third member of the trio.

Empowerment

Embedded within each person is the power to make an improvement. Sometimes this power is lost in the weaknesses, which seem to be more pronounced but look a little closer and you will find at least one strength, which can be a foundation to get better and do something you have always wanted to do.

Empowerment will be irrelevant if we fail to recognize that despite the trauma experiences we can still take the initiative to move our lives in the direction we desire it to go. What do you want to achieve? What do you want your life story to be from this moment on?

Lean into your strength, develop the skills, and get the resources you need to maximize that potential. It may not be possible to do it on your own but it starts with you.

The real you lives within.

UNLOCK YOUR POTENTIAL

It is imperative to have a revelation knowledge of yourself. Not the knowledge of what others tell you about who you are but what you believe you are. Without this, you will be focused on what people know about you on the outside and not who you are on the inside.

This is something I call appearance versus reality. Who you are as a person has very little to do with your outward appearance but everything to do with the inward being. The real you dwell within.

First and foremost, there are so many definitions of human beings. From my understanding derived from my Creator's manual, a human is a Spirit being that has a soul and lives in the body (1 Thessalonians 5:13). I like to look from the dimension that the body is the physical, the soul is the mind while the spirit is the spiritual.

Many train their body to be physically fit, others focus on their soul to be mentally fit while another group focus on the spirit to be spiritually fit. However, many neglect one or more of these components either due to ignorance or the many excuses we all have.

The body can be trained to do certain things but there will be a limitation to commit to it without the accordance of the spirit.

Also, you could go a step further to involve the mind but still without the proper guidance from the spirit the result will be short lived. There is a limit to what physical and mental capacity can produce.

However, whatever is registered in the spirit, what some people call the subconscious mind will automatically influence the mind (conscious mind) and the body. A habit flows from the inside out and not the other way around, which is outside in.

In honesty, most of us will admit that in moments where we felt powerless, we have turned to various substances and activities to fill the longing for a greater power within us. Some have turned to occultism, others to religion, alcohol, drugs and food, yet the longing still lingers. The reason for this is simple, you cannot take a fish out of water and put it on a bed; even a bed made of gold and expects it to thrive.

The moment humans are disconnected from their source, irrespective of the heights and depths of status, wealth and achievements which have been attained, there will always be a feeling that something is missing. There will be a quest to get something but never reaching the full potential.

In order to fully discover our potential, we have to reconnect to our source through a relationship. Personally, I am a daughter of God. Others claim various sources. I cannot say this for other sources because I don't have knowledge of them but I can boldly say this of every child of God through Jesus Christ:

You are powerful, favored, blessed, wise, great, beloved child of God, and you can do whatever you think or imagine because you are strengthened by Christ and through His Spirit living in you, which directs you in the right path. All you need to do is ask, receive and take action!

Know Your World

> The world was not made to encourage you to be your best, but to challenge you to discover what you are capable of doing.

An improper knowledge of the world in which we live will repress your potential rather than aid you in discovering all you can be. A failure to understand this has caused frustration and disappointments to set in the lives of many aiming to move higher on the ladder of recovery and success.

The world was not made to encourage you to be your best, but to challenge you to discover what you are capable of doing. I look at the world as a marketplace. It is a very competitive market because everyone has something to sell though very few have discovered the product they have to offer.

Unless you discover how you fit into the marketplace, you will continue selling counterfeit products. I love this quote by Maya Angelou, "If you are always trying to be normal, you will never know how amazing you can be."

What society considers normal today is something that was discovered by another person years ago and because it has been celebrated so much and accepted as the norm, it has become the standard. I bet you, it was not so when it was first introduced into the marketplace.

The Leader in You

Everyone was made to have dominion on the earth. You are a leader at something but because you turned to the world to tell you the area of your leadership, you have become a servant and not a leader.

The word dominion sounds like a heavy word, especially to some us who have experienced various forms of abuse – political, physical, emotional, cultural, or religious. This is because people are constantly trying to have dominion over others, so as a result they have caused chaos and wars in others and in the world.

You were made to dominate with an idea and not dominate people. You dominate in the idea you discovered in order to serve people. The most renowned people who have exercised control over the world today are not the dictators who tried to suppress the people with their position of influence but those who discovered an idea, stretched it to its full potential until it is known in the four corners of the Earth.

Do not look into the world, look into yourself to make discoveries of your potential. I know your internal perception may be tinted with the lies the world through your abusers may have told you but I tell you today it is time to get another opinion of yourself. Others might lead you to it but the answer rests within you.

Don't put your destiny in the hands of another person; it is time for you to create the life you want and you deserve. This might seem risky to you but some risks are worth taking.

There is an African proverb that says, "If there is no enemy within the enemy outside can do no harm." If you are not willing to take the risk then you are working with the enemy outside to prevent you from growing, and if you can't grow, you can't become your best and if you can't be your best, you can never know all you are capable of doing.

> "You have to be willing to get outside your comfort zone." —Norman Vincent Peale

Take responsibility for your life. You have all the resources you need to get what you are worth. My prayer is that this book will be one of those resources to help break some barriers and assist you on your journey to a personally satisfying life.

JOURNEY WITH KIKI

Kiki came from an area where it was frightening to show any kind of mental weakness. She had seen many lives plagued with stigma. It was enough to make her shun from any complaints regarding her mental wellness.

Added to that, she had never come in contact or even heard of a strength-based approach, which saw the value in every person irrespective of their challenges. All she was familiar with was judgment and discrimination.

She had dreaded the day of her initial appointment with the organization. Thanks to her newfound friend who offered to pick her up and accompany her to the appointment, she had somewhat less hesitation about showing up for it.

At the end of the day, she was glad she went. Not only did she feel comfortable, accepted and relaxed, for the greater part of her meeting, she also experienced genuine interest in her well-being. At her discretion, she was assigned a buddy to check in with her periodically and support her with her necessary needs and resources.

REFLECTION

1. What is your experience with trauma?
2. Is Recovery possible and why?
3. Are you hopeful? What is the source/focus of your hope?
4. If you could only accomplish one thing from this point on in your life, what will it be?
5. Do you feel empowered? What can you do to increase your empowerment?

CHAPTER 2:
YOU MATTER

"Owning our story and loving ourselves through the process is the bravest thing we'll ever do." —*Brené Brown*

Torn apart by the circumstances of life; broken by the challenges within and without; reaching out to a troubled world for answers; driven deeper into the drain of despair! It seems this is all there is to life, these feelings are at constant battle. I hear them say there is a light at the end of the tunnel. How do I get there? There is not an ounce of energy to push on any further. Staying in the middle seems to be the solution right now, for the last strength was drowned in the last!

It is often said that time heals all wounds but that doesn't seem to be true for some of us. The years have gone by but time seems to have passed without its healing power.

Scanning through the room one day, one can hardly miss the beautiful portrait of a young girl with the most beautiful baby. If only the priceless smiles on the face of that mother in the picture could permanently wash away the scenes from a childhood of abuse, pain and losses which ushered her into the stage of a teenager as a mother. The memories of the past never seem to go away. There is an emptiness within, which cannot be filled with any new encounters. When the gap in that hole expresses its loneliness, all substitutes for filing it prove abortive.

THE COVER-UP

So very often we speak so many words to cover up for the pain we feel on the inside. Besides words, we use other media to cover up. We may all be very familiar (especially women) with the extra lengths we go to cover things on the outside of our bodies.

The beach cover dress we wear to cover our bikinis, which we are still debating if we should have worn, the hat we wear to cover messy hair we didn't get a chance to wash or do. I was not about to leave out the corset, Spanx, waist trainer depending on what you choose to call it, which we use to tuck in the extra body fat we're trying to hide and of course the layers of make-up we assume will cover up some oily skin or fine, smile, and aging lines.

> **What we don't realize is that internal covering costs us so much emotional energy.**

We go through so much conscious effort to achieve outside covering but with so little effort we have covered lots of emotions within us. In some cases, it is as easy as saying, "I don't want to talk about that." That lone statement has caused more havoc than you can imagine. What we don't realize is that internal covering costs us so much emotional energy.

With outside covering we do so much for our "secret" to stay hidden. However, with internal covering we don't do the things we should that will relieve us from concealed baggage. The thing with covering up is that after a while it will eventually spill, leaving us with more pain than coming plain.

It is like the make-up we wear, after going through all the effort to cover up something on our face, we need a make-up remover to get it off each day we use it. Failure to do so will result in clogged pores, breakouts, pimples or some other skin defect. The internal covering up we have failed to remove has cost us meaningful relationships, and the chance to enjoy greater joy.

Listen to this voice right now telling you, it is time to stop covering up and seek a change.

It is time to go through that process to change from the inside out.

Internal coverings can keep us away from so much we want to do and can do. You cannot continue to go on like that anymore. You need the change not for anyone in your life – but for you.

Invite honesty into the picture for an inventory, and you will realize that there is something within you, for your benefit, which will eventually overflow to the world.

The change will not come in an instant. It is a process. It is time to go through that process to change from the inside out.

… the journey of recovery has to start with you.

How often do we harbor the guilt when others hurt us? I don't know about you but I have blamed myself for some of the hurtful experiences I have encountered though technically I didn't invite them to happen to me.

It is easier for me to penalize me for your behavior because in my opinion I have control over me but not over the person who hurt me. This is why when we are hurt we choose to stock our bodies with substances: alcohol, food and drugs because most of our trauma sources involve something getting into us so we tend to develop a coping mechanism; in order to deal with this trigger I have to put more stuff in the inside. Often at this time, the thoughts which circulate the mind time after time is, "It is my body; at least I can do whatever I want with it."

How many of you will agree with me that this helps for the first seconds but comes back accompanied by guilt or shame. I find that the most lasting way to exercise my control over me is to control what comes out of me and not what goes into me. Perhaps this is because trauma deposited something inside so in order to relieve it I have to bring out something from within me, something that empowers me, some words of truth to erase the lies.

It often turns out that words have more power than I can explain because when these positive words of affirmation come out, they often bring a control over what is allowed to go into me. The reason could be that when there is peace and stillness within, it attracts from the outside the things and people that will multiply the peace and stillness. It cannot happen when you are upset with yourself.

> ... the requirement of that oneness is for you to love and forgive you.

Don't be alarmed if you are not in that position. The solution to getting to that state is being one with you. Victory does not come by fighting against your own self. Therefore the requirement of that oneness is for you to love and forgive you.

This may not be what we have been told. We are often told to forgive and love others, but I believe it has to start with you. Come to think of it, you can never give out what you don't have. Love and forgiveness can only genuinely flow from you if you have embraced it personally.

WHY YOU HAVE TO FORGIVE YOURSELF

You are human

You can be the best at what you do but you are not perfect. Why do I say so? Every time you go through a work of art you just made – painting, writing, acting, singing or whatever you love to do – you will always find something you could have done differently or at least I always do.

I may have received a 100 percent grading for the art but deep down I know there is something which, if altered, will improve the art. Life is not mathematics, meaning if you follow the formula you will always end with the perfect result. Life is spontaneous – that is what makes us human and not robots.

You may not like this but it is best to know that outcomes will not always be in accordance to your plan. Accept this truth so you can forgive and love yourself.

Stop tormenting yourself for the things you are telling yourself would have happened if you had done something differently. You could be holding forgiveness from yourself because to you, if you didn't use that path or leave the house at that time you would not have been raped. You could also have believed your accuser who said if you didn't dress in a mini skirt you would not have invited him to sexually abuse you. You cannot be exactly sure of that so drop it and move on.

I have also met adults of childhood domestic violence who are still living with the guilt that they are the reason for their parents' fights, sickness or death of a parent. You may not have been an ideal child; that is if there are any, but you don't know all the emotional, physical, medical or spiritual problems your parents had. I am certain your action was nothing compared to their problems.

We may not be proud of the things that happened to us and could wish our experiences were different but we also have to acknowledge that our role is limited.

The best you can do for yourself is to release your destiny, future and life through forgiving and loving yourself.

Irreplaceable

You may have heard someone say you are unique, you are a masterpiece. Part of being unique means you have seeds of greatness within you, which only you can cultivate. Your environment, which is your upbringing, might play a role in this cultivation process but there is an amount of work that requires your action.

Your abusers may have told you otherwise: like you will never turn out to be anything meaningful in life; you are worthless, or you are a failure. Do yourself a favor by not listening to them. People often speak as a result of their own dysfunction. Do not allow your seed to be killed by their toxins.

Unless you forgive and love yourself, you will never see those seeds of greatness so they will never be cultivated.

What hatred and unforgiveness do is that they act as filth, which buries a portion of you. Each time you think of that grudge and dwell on it, you throw filth on your seed. You can turn that filth to fertilizer by changing the grudge to love.

The scenes of torture, violence and abuse may cause you to want to settle where you are; please don't give in. The world needs that uniqueness, which only you can bring into it. You are the only you that will ever exist in this world.

For you to have gone through all those experiences and still be here today is an indication that your best days are still ahead of you. Don't give up now! Don't underrate what you possess because of the lies you have believed. Let go of yourself to embrace yourself.

Give an example

Give what you want. You could call it reaping what you sow but in the context of love and forgiveness, when you give this to yourself, it produces goodness. Yay! Who doesn't want to be around goodness? People and things want to come to something good because goodness is comparable to value so out of goodness flows value.

One of the best gifts you can give the world is an example of how to love you and what forgiveness means to you. The best way I know to do this is to demonstrate to them by the way you do it to yourself. Many of us have searched or are still searching for people to love us. We seek others to forgive us where we have erred.

Most people, whether they recognize it or not are looking for one thing – love. We are in a search of who or what to love and who or what to love us back. Are we going to recognize what we seek if it stands in our presence?

It is also in our human nature to tend to accept only what we can recognize. If I come to you and tell you I love you, it probably won't mean much to you. But if you see how much I love myself, it might move you to want me to extend that love to you.

You cannot make a meaningful improvement on yourself if you haven't first accepted who you are.

Love and forgiveness extended to yourself is a demonstration that you have accepted yourself. The reason self-acceptance is important is that you cannot make a meaningful improvement on yourself if you haven't first accepted who you are.

Also, self-acceptance opens the door for others to accept you. It might not be so obvious to you but you will never accept that someone loves you, someone has forgiven you or someone has accepted you if you have not first offered yourself that opportunity to demonstrate it to you. The prerequisite to identify these qualities is to first offer it to ourselves so that when you tell someone 'I love and forgive you', you are thereby saying 'I love and forgive you in the same way I love and forgive myself'.

Contrary to what you may have known, self-love is not selfish; it is a demonstration of what you have and what you can offer to others.

Relieves the pain

According to Dr. Susanne Babbel, a somatic psychologist, "Studies have shown that chronic pain might not only be caused by physical injury but also by stress and emotional issues."[3] I totally relate to this because so much stress emanates from asking the question, "How could I have…?" Whatever comes after the question mark is an indication of taking the shame for something that didn't go in the perceived direction.

There are times we experience pain from injuries but some of us can relate to pain in the absence of any physical justification. If you have been there like me, you can attest that it is not where we want to be at any point in time.

Personally and with confirmation from some lovely people who shared their story with me, this pain stems from an overwhelming challenge to deal with inner conflicts.

Often, we strive to resolve conflicts with others but fail to resolve it with ourselves. If you have to truly resolve a conflict you have to begin with yourself. This is because somewhere within you there is a reason why you take responsibility for that conflict. It might be true or imaginary but it doesn't take our mind off our role in it.

In resolving it, first identify that part where you think you are at fault. Then forgive yourself for it so you can let go of that pain.

If I come to you saying 'I forgive you' when I have not forgiven myself, I am only deceiving myself because when my alleged role in the problem comes to mind, not only will I be angry at myself, roll it over to you internally, but I will feel the pain from the turmoil within.

To get rid of this pain and the chances of it occurring due to a specific problem; notice I said specific because it could come up as a result of another problem but to get rid of it in this specific problem, I have to first forgive myself so I can forgive you with joy from within.

Joy doesn't mean I am happy to forgive you because often we are not happy to forgive our offenders. Joy means I am at a position of peace with myself to let go of your offense towards me.

A purpose

There is a difference between something happening to you on purpose and you having a purpose. It is important to make that clarification because not too long ago, it came up while I was talking to a trauma thriver. She explained to me the anger she feels when someone tells her there is a purpose for the abuse she experienced earlier in her life.

To her, giving a purpose to her experience is giving her abusers the victory in the situation. It is saying if she had not encountered that experience she wouldn't have had a specific outcome. To her that thought is hurtful and re-traumatizing. I validate her thoughts because we all have diverse triggers to trauma.

> What I know for sure is that there is a purpose for you being alive.

My response to her is what I am telling you now. There could be a purpose for that, which we do not know about. However what I know for sure is that there is a purpose for you being alive. It could have a connection to the experience or not, that is left for you to discover.

In my opinion, the abusers are only given the victory and power to re-traumatize you when you refuse to give yourself love and forgiveness. In this case, you are allowing their act to pull you back from discovering and/or fully engaging in your purpose.

HOW DO I MOVE ON?

You are valuable, you matter, you are important, but it doesn't end with you. There is much more to your existence than yourself. In order to experience all that can flow out of you, all the energy you can bring into the world and all the services you can provide to make your world a better place, you have to be willing to move on through these practical steps.

Step 1: Own Your Story

Our story is very important in liberating ourselves into the future we deserve. It gives us the opportunity to question our beliefs, examine our fears, straighten the facts, identify the lies, replace them with the truth and rewrite the story with our desired outcome.

Reclaiming our story gives us the chance to call in our inner power to defeat the words our abusers may have chiselled into us; words of lack translated through "I am not good enough," "I am not worthy." You can rewrite it with the truth of who you are.

Step 2: Monitor Your Thoughts

When you choose to own your story it is vital to monitor the thoughts that flow into your mind. Like many people with trauma experiences, there may be a template of fear, which you have to get rid of and replace with courage, faith and positivity. It may not be the position you are in now but it is imperative to practice typing in good thoughts about yourself into your mind through self-talk also known as autosuggestion.

Another way is to do the best you can to bring your thoughts into the present. If you are now in a safe physical environment; away from the source of trauma, you can start by calming your mind by telling it you are safe now each time it drifts to the past.

Talking to your mind is a way of taking authority over your body, something which sadly many of us did not have to privilege to at some point in our lives. Now you have the power to take authority over your body through your thoughts by making a choice of how you want to feel and react in the present moment and the future.

Step 3: Don't Personalize
Recognize that you are not the sole creator of the choices of others; if you have a role in influencing their choices it is probably insignificant. Have you ever heard of the saying, "Hurting people hurt others?" While I am not making excuses for the wrong that was done to you, do not take the actions of others personally. As diverse as the people walking on the streets are, so are the issues they are dealing with.

Step 4: Practice
There can never be too much emphasis laid in practicing self-love and wellness. No one may be able to give you this, so it is something you owe to yourself.

JOURNEY WITH KIKI

Kiki is very familiar with the Bible phrase "…Love your neighbor as yourself…" (Mark 12:31). The shortcoming is that she was so focused on the first part of it she didn't pay much attention to the latter part of the statement at least in practice.

Being the oldest among her siblings she was primed to nurture and care for them. She gently extended this character to everyone she came across without giving much attention to deliberately taking care of her own physical, emotional, and/or spiritual health.

She always disregarded her own needs until her well-being came to a point of breakdown. In her moment of exhaustion, she began to feel despised, like her efforts didn't matter anymore by the people whose needs she once placed before hers.

The emotions of hopelessness, fear, shame, anger, and sadness became too overwhelming for her to bear. As if that was not enough, she began to experience excruciating pain in her chest, unresponsiveness, difficulties falling and staying asleep as well as extreme fatigue.

From her new circle of friends, she learned that part of her recovery process will entail healthy self-care. Contrary to her belief, she came to the knowledge that taking care of yourself is not selfishness but a priority.

It was a huge blessing for her to have her buddy who without judgement would express opinions when her self-care cup seemed to require refilling.

Kiki was amazed at how "little things" like deep breaths, smiling at herself in the mirror, short walks and talking to a friend made a huge difference in her well-being.

REFLECTION

1. How did you feel when you tried to cover up a pain? What did you do to release that feeling?
2. Is there any area in your life that you need to forgive yourself?
3. Can you really give out forgiveness and love without bitterness if you haven't forgiven and loved yourself?
4. How do you show yourself some love?
5. What are some yellow lights to show that your self-love tank needs refilling? How do you refill it?

CHAPTER 3:
PLUG IN

"You can't be an important and life-changing presence for some people without also being a joke and an embarrassment to others." —*Mark Manson*

FINDING YOUR TRIBE

Recently, I hear a lot of people talking about finding your tribe. The first time I heard this, it made me laugh because my initial thought was, "What do they mean by finding your tribe or I am looking for my tribe?" Don't get me wrong, my laughter was not geared towards the people saying it but from my knowledge of tribe shaped by the environment where I was born and first nurtured.

That knowledge says a tribe is a something that happens naturally, you didn't ask for it, you didn't look for it, you just happen to be part of it by the nature of your birth. That is why I call it a natural tribe. It never occurred to me or anyone I knew of as something you have to find. It is so natural that someone you meet for the first time will be able to identify your tribe from your name. If the person happens to be more knowledgeable about your tribe, they could go the extra mile of identifying your family by your name.

So I began reflecting on what is this whole notion of finding your tribe. Then it dawned on me that most sources of trauma often emanate from the members of a person's natural tribe. Particularly in communities that have not experienced much emigration or immigration.

Often abuse has come from family members, neighbors or someone who is closely related in one way or another, i.e. a person you will often consider to be a member of your tribe. A good number of people can relate to trauma from cultural practices because their natural tribe requires them to undergo that particular ritual. Others did not end up in a union with a person they connected with because they come from different natural tribes. So, is it better to stick to your natural tribe or find one?

> For healing or recovery from trauma to fully take place, the individual has to be in a safe environment.

Today, I who once laughed at the finding your tribe movement have become an advocate for it because for healing or recovery from trauma to fully take place, the individual has to be in a safe environment. First, it has to be safe physically and secondly, it has to be safe emotionally.

More harm is always done when we seek help in the wrong places. A natural tribe could be the place where the greatest judgements and shaming takes place so that is definitely not your tribe for recovery. You need a tribe of like-minded individuals to support your recovery journey. A tribe that suits your goals, tunes your vision and suitable for your purpose.

In other words, a trauma recovery tribe has to be one of commonality that goes beyond your blood type or family history. A place of connection, a place of support and a place for growth, a place where you can finally say, "This is where I belong!"

However, finding your tribe is just the first step, there is more to come.

Some cultures may be very supportive of letting out emotions in times of and after adversity but sadly most of our cultures advocate for the opposite.

VULNERABILITY! REALLY?

Those who are honest with themselves will admit that we all go through life with some internal pain though most of us try to make everyone around us think we have everything in order in our lives for one reason or another. Some can trace this to fear of shame or stigma. Most of us can't really explain why we choose to hide our hurts. The silliness of life is that we are all hiding our hurts from people who are also hurting yet they too are struggling to shield theirs.

Within every human is deposited the longing to belong. Admit it or not, there is a burning desire in each person walking the earth to have some kind of connection to the world outside them. Along with belongingness comes vulnerability. While we want to belong, we do not want to come across as being vulnerable so we choose not to expose a portion of ourselves even to the people that matter most to us.

> **In order to fully embrace yourself and be all that you can be, you must embrace vulnerability.**

We dread the outcome of exposing our pain because we want to connect with others, we want relationships to be lasting or at least for us to receive what we expect from others. Because, somewhere deep within us, there is that belief that the more the other party knows who we are for real, the greater the chances of a failed relationship.

Everyone on earth has a story not visible on their faces for all to read. Everybody is dealing with something which when you come to that realization, you honestly do not have to wear a mask to impress people who have their own struggles.

In order to fully embrace yourself and be all that you can be, you must embrace vulnerability. The more we hide our most painful experiences, the greater the chances of us feeling unworthy thereby walking around with a lack of confidence in ourselves and abilities.

In case you are wondering what vulnerability means, this definition from Oprah Winfrey on the *Living Brave with Brené Brown* show put it across to me. She said, "[Vulnerability is] being willing to express the truth no matter what, the truth of who you are, the essence at your core, what you are feeling at any given moment. It is being able to open up your soul and let it flow so that other people can see their soul in yours."[4]

That is very deep because how many of us are truly willing to open up our flaws and let the real us flow through? Some have turned to various substances, actions and adopt a certain lifestyle to suppress the story and prevent being vulnerable. As many as the maladaptive strategies are, so are the numerous stories of failed attempts to numb the story. In desperation and dire need, many do not know who or what to turn to because most of us look at vulnerability as a weakness as opposed to the strength it really is.

TRUST AND BETRAYAL

It is clearly visible that the relationships in our lives seem so superficial that we don't know who to believe, trust, and rely on. There is a lot of pretense walking down the street because no one wants to talk about the real issues they should be talking about. Would you blame them? Perhaps not! Not all that glitters is gold so the fact that someone smiles at you or happens to be a close relation doesn't make them a candidate to access the deepest issues in your heart.

Sincerely, many of us do not want to be open about our painful experiences because we don't know who to trust. The moment you open your mouth to talk to someone you think you trust could be the same moment you open up yourself to betrayal.

The process of being vulnerable is a gradual one.

Trust and betrayal go hand in hand. At the same moment, if you do not get or give one, you get or give the other. The process of being vulnerable is a gradual one. If you want to be open about your deepest pain and not get betrayed be open to someone who says what they will do and do it over and over all the time – a person of integrity and reliability.

Personally, I can only share my painful experiences with someone I don't trust when that experience is no longer a pain to me. In other words, I can walk up to you, lay out a part of my heart to you when that part has been healed so it doesn't matter if you explain it to the person sitting right next to you as soon as I turn my back.

The reason I am a person of faith is because I choose to have someone I can trust. A person I know who says what he will do and do it over and over and over again, every word of his always turns out to be true. That makes him the most reliable person I can count on.

If you are like me who was raised in a household of faith, you will probably attest to the fact that coming from that background didn't automatically provide all the answers you need to some of the difficult experiences you have encountered. It doesn't automatically put you in the position to trust a power greater than you.

It is even more common for people like us from that upbringing to come across as "having it all together," which sincerely makes it hard for others to relate with us the way they really want to. This often emanates from an image of always being strong and painless, which is not the reality. If everything is really going in order then we really don't need God or whatever you consider to be your source of faith.

In my case, the God I know is looking for the real you, to take away your burden and give you His rest. That too means I can be vulnerable to Him, and He will direct me on what steps to take, who to open up to and from experience that always comes with an inner peace, which is what I want to feel when I release the deepest secrets of my heart.

If you don't want to be come across as being vulnerable before humans, take a chance to be vulnerable before your source by exposing your hurts, your pains to Him or what you choose to address your higher power and if need be, you will be led to those who can help you heal.

Be vulnerable with real people who will strengthen you through your trial. Be open to a trusted friend who has earned the right to hear your honesty if you have any.

In my early years, I came to understand that being strong means bearing your burdens alone, acting up in front of people and crying in your closet.

Be honest with yourself and with the person(s) who understand your difficult moments, sees your struggle but wants your humility by you admitting your hard moments so you can be helped to overcome what you truly will never be able to overcome on your own.

I NEED YOU

Don't try to get it all together on your own. Don't try to clean up the mess by yourself whether you created it or were dragged into it. It takes so much more than you can imagine, but there is someone waiting to walk you through; to get you out of the unfavorable situation.

Most of us have mistaken positivity to mean 'I can do it all by myself.' In reality, being positive means despite what I am going through things will not always be like this; there is a light at the end of the tunnel. Being vulnerable is looking up towards that light.

There comes a time to expose your wounds to fully heal.

While being positive to overcome that stage, don't hide your hurts. Wounded flesh will not fully heal if it is always covered. In fact, it could get worse and gross if not exposed to some sunlight. There comes a time to expose your wounds to fully heal.

We all need one another; you can never know who needs you if you don't open up. If you are not open, you cannot know those who are waiting for you so they can get their healing. Everyone is a part of a puzzle. You have to spread the pieces of your bruises in order to fit your piece into another person's piece to create a portion of the whole.

One of the lessons I have learned as a parent is that my children learn more from me when they see the sincerity in my words and action. There was once I made a mistake, not the first but one of them (which I am sure every parent will admit to doing a couple a day), my daughter who was four years old at the time said, "Mommy, you made a mistake. It's okay. Everyone makes mistakes. Try to fix it and learn from it." I am sure you know how bitter it is to swallow a pill prescribed by you.

I have been teaching this to her in theory but it comes alive in practice when she gets the opportunity to demonstrate the theory. Let the people in your life see the real you so they can appreciate you more when they see how you are being molded into a new vessel.

I have come across many people from various ethnicities hurting in their relationships because their partners were raised to believe and practice that a strong human doesn't have to reveal their pains, hurts and weaknesses because that is for weaklings. From observation, the irony is that most of these partners end up expressing anger, resentfulness towards the very people who should not be at the receiving end of these reactions.

Holding on to the pain as opposed to not wanting to come across as vulnerable results in dealing with hidden issues in unhealthy ways, which affects many relationships. Is it better to expose your pain and receive healing than seek solace in ways you are not proud of? The ball is in your court.

There is something in the humility of not being driven by what anyone else says but allowing yourself to lay out your pain and take hold of your healing. Traditions, cultures, religions have told us we are real men, independent women if we swallow our hurts and move on like nothing ever happened. But, there comes a time in life when you realize the mask doesn't work anymore. It covers the wounds to the outside but doesn't stop the maggots from digging at the wound on the inside, making it worse, bigger and stinky to the bearer. Ultimately, it becomes a stench the bearer has become accustomed to but the same people the wound is being covered from can smell it when you come around them.

> The fact that you do not admit something doesn't make it go away. The first step in a healing process is to acknowledge that there is a problem; the pain exists.

I encourage you today not to hide your shortcomings; do not push back your painful past and present experiences. The fact that you do not admit something doesn't make it go away. The first step in a healing process is to acknowledge that there is a problem; the pain exists. It is okay to acknowledge your weaknesses and your need for help. Denying the existence of something doesn't make it go away. Let it go!

I write to you about letting it go from experience. Holding on to past hurts, acting like the events never existed only led me to make poor choices, which would have led my life to a direction other than what I desired for myself.

When I decided to expose the contents of my heart to the one who knows me more than anyone else, not only did I get the relief I had been looking for but didn't find in other places, I also received the chance to retrace the course of my life and steer it towards a more favorable destination.

At a point where I felt content that I was having the things I always wanted but felt I could never have a chance to experience because I once thought my life was over, I said to myself that the painful portion of my past is over. I will never talk about it, never share it and move on it like it never happened.

With my mind settled on this point though I was still not at peace. The voice of wisdom whispered to me: "I want you to disclose your wounds so you can bring healing to others." Today. I choose to be a peer because I realize that there are people at different points in their journey who need a buddy to walk with them for the release from their cage.

Once buckled in, I find it a fascinating miracle each time I share a slice of my life with others because as many people as I talk to I get the satisfaction that someone somewhere needs to know there is much more to their lives than their circumstances. You are not destined to drown in abuse, betrayal, trauma and hardship.

> *With your consent, your life can be unlocked to reveal a whole new horizon.*

JOURNEY WITH KIKI

Being in a safe tribe ultimately gave Kiki the confidence to open up about her past. It didn't happen in a day, a week or a month but at a time when she felt emotionally ready to seek support. On that fateful day, in her safe place, she went on to say:

Traveling down memory lane, this course of my life started when I was about six years old. Life in my remarkable rural city was full of fun for an adventurous kid. Obviously, that adventurous part of me was subdued at some point. There were no fancy playgrounds, amusement parks, zoos or aquariums to visit, but there were lots of natural undeveloped beaches at the river banks that also serve as a bathroom for baths and laundry room for the inhabitants of the city.

Some of these rivers were also highly commercial avenues for travellers to and from the neighboring countries coming to them mostly by boat, they were a source of income for those who import and export goods and touristic sites for the few tourists who dared to travel the muddy, untarred difficult road to get to the beautiful city whose contents are worth the sacrifice.

It was always fun to play in the sand with the other children whom you may be meeting for the first time and may never meet again. In most cases, you might meet other children from your school or the kids next door considering it was a city of a few thousand people.

This wasn't the only play place for children in this metropolitan milieu. Like it was everywhere else in the country, children regularly meet outside in the neighborhood to play various impromptu games or a well-defined game like hopscotch, skip rope or hide and seek. While the girls were busy spending energy with these activities, the boys often had other plans. You could find the guys playing football for fun or practicing with the hope of fulfilling their dreams of becoming a renowned football player.

They may not have known how much money the celebrity footballers make but they did know they were the envy of every young man. Besides the money, who didn't want to be a household name in the nation or make every onlooker the next possible candidate for a heart attack if you miss a goal?

Though the boys and girls had their games cut out, they would sometimes come together to play a game like hide and seek, which all the children enjoyed. The children all buzzed around enjoying their games mostly without adult supervision. It was a time for adults to focus on chores, rest, chatting without constant interruptions from children.

Kiki paused for a long minute and went on to say:

One beautiful day, we happened to be playing a game of hide and seek. When my turn to hide came around, I searched for a hidden spot to smuggle my little self. It was small enough for me to fit in and big enough not to be seen. Never did I imagine that it would turn out to be a spot where a fellow player who later showed up asking to share a hideout would later touch me inappropriately.

Leaving the hiding place in tears, which emanated from being called horrible names by someone who felt he had the right to do what he did and I had no right to protest verbally, it looked relieving to recount the incident to the first third person I saw who happened to be a relative to my offender, precisely his big brother.

To my dismay, the protective older sibling called the incident child's play and vehemently warned me not to let any other ear hear about the incident, especially my parents. He went on to say if I told someone, the next hearer will call me a bad child, and I will be punished severely for what just happened.

My little six-year-old brain believed the thirteen-year-old big brother who to me was wiser and smarter. He asked me to wipe my tears, go home and act like nothing ever happened. Being the obedient kid in the block, I followed every detail of his plan. No one ever suspected I had encountered such an incident but the effect of my silence didn't remain silent considering it didn't wait too long to make itself loud.

Two years after, my loving parents came to have a talk with me just before bedtime. With doubts in my heart as to what I may have done to deserve this unusual visit, I sat down patiently waiting for them to start the conversation. My dear father went on to state the purpose of the meeting. "Kiki," he said, "we have come to let you know that according to our tradition, you are now of age to be introduced into womanhood. The introduction of you being a woman requires that you will be circumcised."

While I was still trying to make meaning out of the words I just heard, my mother went on to say, "My dear daughter, what your father is saying is not something new. I went through it and every woman in our family has to go through it. Tomorrow your aunt will come get you in the morning. She will bring you back to us as a woman."

I was confused and anxious, not knowing what to expect the next day. Was it going to be a fun game? What exactly is going to happen to me? The questions kept spinning in my head until I fell as sleep just to wake up to the D-day.

As promised, my aunt was at my house by 5:00 a.m. the following day. She said we had to leave as soon as possible because the rite had to be performed before sunrise in order to prevent excessive bleeding. I asked who was going to bleed and why but the response I got was "Everything is going to be okay."

My aunt took me into a hut where other women and children were waiting for our arrival. The other girls and I were made to take off our clothes and tie a loincloth across our chest with no under clothes. We were blindfolded and tied with the reason that the place where the rite will take place is very sacred so we children are not allowed to see the route that leads to it.

We were led into the "sacred place". All of a sudden I heard drumming and singing in our native language. I could identify the language because my grandparents spoke it occasionally to me though I didn't understand it because I didn't hear it often. At that moment, all I wished for was to understand the language so it could give me insight into what was happening or about to happen.

After what seemed like an eternity, the blindfold was taken off my eyes. It appears it was my turn, for standing in front of me was an elderly woman with a sharp knife and blood dripping from it; perhaps the blood of the other girls whose screams have been filling my heart with fear and pity.

The sight of the lady caused me to fight to free myself, but there was little I could do with my arms tied and four women forcing me to lay on the plantain leaves laid out on the ground. Their strength prevailed as I lay down while one of the ladies covered my mouth, and the lady with the knife went ahead to cut off what I later found out was my clitoris.

The pain and bleeding of the day stayed with me for more than one month while I received "treatment" for the rites. I cried day and night as I looked forward to the day I would be reunited with my parents. After two months, I was finally taken back to my parents. What a joy it was to see them again.

Oh my! Did I know my return was to mark the beginning of another ordeal?

Kiki paused; as she let the tears roll down her cheeks. The leader of her community group said, "You can stop if you are not comfortable to move on." Kiki said, "I will go on. I have buried this for too long, though it is hard I believe it is time to spill it out."

Months after my return, my father called me into his room when my mother was not home. He told me he wanted to examine the work the women had done to ensure it was done properly. That marked the beginning of sexual abuse from my father.

One day, I summoned the courage to tell my mother about it assuming she didn't know since the act always took place when she was away. She didn't act like it was a surprise to her but she went ahead to say I should never tell anyone about it because my father is a respectable man in the community, and it will be very bad for me to ruin his reputation.

In exchange for my silence, pain, and tolerance, my parents lavished me with presents and every material thing I asked from them.

Just when I thought the abuse couldn't get worse, on a day like any other, I was in the neighbors' compound probably to play with the other children my age that lived there. While there, the teenage boy of that family called me into the house and forced himself into me sexually. I don't remember if I was told not to tell anyone about it or if I decided to keep it a secret like I have been told in my early years and by my family but the physical and emotional pain was kept buckled in my heart.

I kind of felt I had to be a faithful servant to the art of silence. Someone out there could have set me free from the pain if I had shared it then or at least prevent the incident from reoccurring. But who could I talk to if my own parents had warned me to be quiet in a similar scenario?

However, my silence may have been interpreted as compliance as from that day onward he would regularly ask his siblings to call me to come play with them and then distract them by sending them on errands so he could perform the deplorable act. The abuse got to the point where I thought this is life for me so I allowed myself to concede into it.

With a head bowed down in shame they must have placed an inscription on it that said, "This child can be sexually violated and she will be silent about it" because one incident just seemed to lead to another.

Here I was a lonely little girl who didn't want to go play with her female neighbors for fear that her brothers will violate her, I couldn't live freely in my home without being scared that my father will creep into my bed while I sleep to sexually exploit me.

Raised up to go to a church every Sunday and also studying at a Christian elementary school, I felt the place I could seek solace in, is the church. There was an after school activity at the church where children were taught Bible stories, memory verses, dances, songs and other activities. In my quest for companions, I decided to join this group.

When I got home from school, oftentimes I would drop my backpack and go out to the group I had joined without the knowledge of my family. I was already accustomed to keeping secrets. Unknown to me, my father had noticed my unavailability at home after school. I had thought everyone was too busy with other things and no one noticed my absence.

One evening, when I returned home from church, I bumped into my father who asked where I had been. Excitedly, I told him I had joined the kids group and that is where I was coming from. My dad who was a Christian but not a regular church-goer was very furious at my response.

He warned me to stay away from the group adding that he will punish me severely if he finds out I go to the group after school. This group had given me so much happiness I tried to explain to him that it was good and I tried to explain the memory verses I had learned, the games, the songs and the dances. This angered him more, and said he will not live to see me go back to that church. This may have been just an expression of anger from a concerned father but my little brain didn't take it that way. As I walked out of the room I murmured to myself that may he never live to see me go there.

The next day of the activity at church, I left the house again despite my father's warning. I checked to make sure he was not home. It turned out he was out at a meeting with my mother. Strangely on this day, I couldn't enjoy the songs, the rhymes, the dance or anything that was done; I was anxiously waiting for the activities to be over so I could go home.

As soon as they were over, I took to my heels running home. From a distance, I could see people gathered in our compound in little groups of two, three or more but I couldn't understand what was happening. I didn't leave that many people in the house when I left, besides why did all the neighbors decide to come to my house on that particular day? I was afraid something bad may have happened.

To confirm my fears, as I got closer my paternal aunt spotted me and ran towards me wailing. She gave me a hug and said my parents had passed away in a ghastly car accident. One thing came to my mind, after my father said he will not live to see me go back to the group and my response was may he not live to see me go there. At that point, my nine-year-old mind concluded that I was responsible for the death of my parents.

This incident, coupled with the abuse I had been through, made me believe bad things are meant to happen to me. I had hoped that my life was going to get better at some point but all I got was the guilt of my parents' death and sudden responsibility to look after my two younger siblings. I stopped attending the group meetings that had brought me so much joy hoping that if I don't go there again my parents would come back to life.

They never came back to life. I always thought there was something in me that attracted the wrong situations; that I could not stop bad things from happening to me even when I tried. My failed attempt to bring my parents back to life told me that I had no control over my life so from that moment on I resolved to leave myself at the mercy of situations without fighting back.

REFLECTION

1. What does 'vulnerability' mean to you?
2. If you had to find your tribe what are the characteristics you would look for to be part of your tribe?
3. Supposing you are to write your story, what will you write?

CHAPTER 4:
RE-CREATION

"Rape on the body of a person more often than not introduces cynicism and there is nothing quite so tragic as a young cynic. Because it means the person has gone from knowing nothing to believing nothing." —*Maya Angelou.*

There is no universally accepted excuse for the abuse that has been perpetrated on you or the situation you found yourself in. Worse still, most of us were woven to think through a pattern we are not proud of. In the recovery journey, the most important aspect to recognize and embrace is a shift in our paradigm.

What is a paradigm shift? Merriam-Webster[5] describes it as: "An important change that happens when the usual way of thinking about or doing something is replaced by a new and different way."

In order to change your future, you have to be willing to change your paradigm – what has been moulded into you from the time of your abuse until this point in your life. I have often heard people say they had no life before their initial trauma because they don't remember what life was for them before that. That might be true for you, but what is also true is that you can take control of how your life will go from now on by taking control of your thoughts. So you can choose to recreate what you want from this moment onward.

When you decide to change your paradigm you have to make a decision to change your mindset every second of your life and from there cultivate it to get better and expand how you want your life to be.

For change to happen, the mindset of the person must change first. The mindset to accommodate any harm being done is the cause of many poor choices made later in life. In my case, Maya Angelou sums up my life at that time because I was transposed "from knowing nothing to believing nothing," this includes believing in my abilities.

As I later figured out, nothing controls the destiny of a person like your mental attitude. You have the power to change your destiny – to change your life. Like my favourite book in the world says, "For as a man thinks in his heart so is he." (Proverbs 23:7). The only proven method to change your history is to reposition your mindset.

Mentality is the driving force for destiny however it is often underrated among people striving to achieve a different result, the thoughts allowed to sow seed in a person will determine the outcome of his or her life.

> You can *choose* how to direct how life unfolds
> after the traumatic incident.

The mind is one of God's greatest gifts to mankind yet it is one of the most neglected areas in the body. Whatever lingers in the mind will bear fruit. The mind is a soil to cultivate the thoughts we plant in it so the fruit can grow out for the world to see. You have to choose the kind of fruit you want to produce. You can *choose* how to direct how life unfolds after the traumatic incident.

I used to think where I am today is solely because God allowed it to be so. As true as it sounds, it is not entirely true. The mind is like a cooking pot, when you decide to cook you put different kinds of ingredients in the pot but the ingredient with the strongest flavour determines the taste of the food. In order words, where we are today is not solely because God made it so but a product of what has been allowed to taste stronger in our minds.

There is a giant deposited within each human being on planet earth. This can either be nurtured to grow with one mindset or suppressed by another. For most people, what their abusers told them caused a suppression of their greatness. It is left on the individual to choose to allow the greatness to stay suppressed or nurture it to grow. Mental set is a choice harnessed with conscious or unconscious discipline. It is not a trait bestowed upon the lucky or the unlucky.

> For most people, what their abusers told them caused a suppression of their greatness.

We live in a world that has conditioned billions of people to believe that things just happen, what I call a dot com generation. That might be true for a few things but for so many others we have to choose and develop our choices else we will not like the results we get.

My life has been shaped by different types of mentalities just as it has been shaped by circumstances and situations. In my quest for change, I had to pinpoint this mindset to either discard or cultivate it in order to have lasting results.

True change needs a sense of direction. It needs a starting point and an endpoint to know if any change occurred.

MENTALITY OF LACK

The mentality of lack will always make you a pauper because if you keep thinking you lack something, you will never realize you have acquired so much nor have something in you so you will continue living like a destitute person.

This mindset of lack arises when there is little or no contentment. You will always think you lack something if you are not contented with what you have. If you are like me, I used to misunderstand content to mean settle where you are, with no dreams, goals and vision. Now I have come to understand that is not what it means. Content refers to being happy with what you have while exercising faith and working towards getting what you desire.

Content means to be happy in your current season and know that just like the weather changes in due time, in a matter of time that season of your life will come to an end and the next season will begin. The way you manage this season will determine how you will enjoy the next season. If you go around this season thinking you lack something you will still go through the next season focused on what you lack.

What we tend to do is to focus on what we lack and desire. For most of us, we are so focused on getting 'it' that we fail to enjoy our present lives. Discontentment is the norm. In other words, contentment doesn't happen automatically, it is the result of a choice. Human nature and information in the world and media are geared towards being happy only after you get a particular thing. However, we are wired to be happy to attract what we hope to receive.

Life will bring trials, trauma, pain, and disappointment. This should not break us but bring out the greatness in us. There is a season for everything. The reason it is called a season is that it is not made to last forever. Get up and face another season; the season of planning to move forward, the season of pursuing; the season of celebration.

Don't miss a great season in your life thinking you lack something and wishing you had it. Enjoy this season without complaining. Be determined to enjoy every second of your day no matter who is sour and bitter around you. See a gift in everything and every situation; see a day as a moment that will never repeat itself. If you lose the chance to enjoy it, you will never have another opportunity to enjoy that same day.

While reading an issue of *Success Magazine*, the writer Aaron Orendorff quoted in *Option B: Facing adversity, building resilience, and finding joy*. He wrote, "Sometimes, life's most painful, unexpected, and tragic experiences can give you something positive. Building your resilience can help you move forward in business and in life."[6]

In the process of losing something, we always gain something. If you look far enough you will get some of it but if you don't look at all you will get nothing. It is your choice to decide if you want the gain to be something beneficial or something destructive. For most people, they gain strength. For those who are still to discover their gains, it is probably covered in the blanket of lack. Take off the blanket, and you will see your gains. You have everything you need to succeed.

VICTIM/VICTOR MENTALITY

Oftentimes, we do not choose every detail of the circumstances we find ourselves in. For some things, it is common to everyone: you don't choose where you are born, the neighbourhood you grow up in, your name at birth, your siblings, and your parents. For others, it goes beyond this into their childhood experiences. Some people just happened to be one of those who had exceptional childhood experiences, which they did nothing to deserve. This has shaped some minds to respond to life from the position of being a target for difficulties.

There are people who have a victim mentality, who think they are prey for toxic people and events while others with a victor mentality think they are conquerors and will conquer every unfavourable situation. You can either have a victim or a victor mentality but hardly both at the same time.

The opinion we have of ourselves matter. It is possible that two people can be in the same location, go through the same situation but produce different results. One emerges successful and the other turns out a failure based on their judgements. Talents, intelligence and strength have very little to do with it, it is all about mental attitude.

Take a close look at the lion and the elephant in the jungle. The lion is known as the king of the animal kingdom whereas the elephant is the largest animal. The elephant is taller than the lion, it is heavier than the lion, it is larger than the lion and probably more intelligent than the lion if we were to do an IQ test. Yet the lion is the king of the jungle and not the elephant, why is that? What makes the lion the king and not the elephant?

The one thing that gives the lion an advantage over the elephant is its mentality; its way of thinking and that is all it needs to be qualified as king over the elephant. When the lion sees the elephant, it thinks of it as food, despite its height, size, knowledge or weight. It goes after it, attacks it and eats it just as it does to a horse, a goat or an ant. To him, no animal is too big for him to conquer or too small to miss. In other words, no problem is unsuitable to overcome.

On the other hand, when the elephant sees the lion, it thinks of it as a consumer and itself as an object for consumption so instead of facing the challenge of the elephant, it tries to run away from it. What this means is that the lion has the mentality of the victor while the elephant has the victim mentality. From the standpoint of the victor, the lion goes ahead to take its victory over the elephant while the elephant from the position of victim runs away from its conqueror.

Your past is not a determinant for the future you deserve.

It is very common to see people with a victim mentality because many believe they are victims of circumstances, victims of politics, victims of the economy, or victims of the social structure. Some people due to no fault of theirs were born into some dysfunctional situations such as abuse, addictions, diseases and neglect. However, do not allow what happened to you cause damage in you. Your past is not a determinant for the future you deserve.

We have become so accustomed to the events of our past that we cannot see what is out there waiting for us to receive. Even when victory stands in front of us we often don't recognize it because it doesn't always come in the package we expect.

Perception and Realities

I once heard the story of a young man who had been admiring a specific sports car for a very long time. He was the only son of a very wealthy man. As his graduation from college was approaching, he asked his father for this car as his graduation gift. He kept looking for signs that his father had purchased this car as the days towards his graduation came closer but he saw no signs. Finally, on the morning after his graduation, his father called him into his home office and told him how proud he was of his achievement. He then handed his son a beautifully wrapped gift box.

Filled with joy and expectation, the son opened this gift and found a lovely leather Bible in a box. With joy turned to rage, he yelled at his father saying, "With all the money you have, can you only afford to give me a Bible? I could buy that if I needed one." He threw the Bible at his father and stomped out of the house.

Several years went by. The young man had no contact with his father; he had obtained a job at a company. He worked hard to pay his bills and meet his needs and have a great future without assistance from his father. One day on his way back from work, he thought of his father. He decided it was time to visit his father since he had not seen him since the incident on his graduation day.

While he was preparing to go see his father, he received a phone call. The caller said his father had passed away, leaving all his possessions to him.

Filled with sadness as he entered his father's home office where he last saw him, he began going through his father's library with nostalgia. He came across the lovely leather Bible he had received as his college graduation gift.

As tears began streaming through his eyes, he flipped through the pages of the Bible. Suddenly, a car key with a tag fell from the Bible. The tag had the name of the same dealer who owned the shop where he had admired his dream sports car. On the tag was inscribed the date of his graduation and below it the words "Paid in full." The young man couldn't control his tears as they streamed down his eyes.

The perception of seeing ourselves as victims and complaining about the situations we have been through prevents us from seeing the victorious life that lies ahead of us. Therefore, whatever we have been through or are going through should not be the basis upon which we judge the outcome of our lives.

> Focus on what you can do for yourself and *not* what others have done to you.

- The first thing you need to do to move from a victim mentality to a victor mentality is to stop seeing yourself from your current perception and see yourself the way you were originally created: a talented, strong, creative, well able and wonderfully made person.
- The second leap to move from the victim to the victor mentality is to begin to focus on what you can do for yourself and not what others have done to you. The change will not occur overnight but it is a great step. With the victim mentality, we give the power over our lives to others while with the victor mentality, we possess the power.

SLAVE MENTALITY

This is a close associate of the victim mentality. A person can operate under either one or a combination of both. For the new generation people who may not have heard the word slaves on social media or studied it in schools like I did, let me explain a little about it so we all can be on the same page.

When we talk about slaves, a person familiar with the word might first think of the slaves in America and Europe beginning in the 1700s or the Israelites as slaves in Egypt as recorded in the books of Genesis and Exodus of the Bible. Those are the two outstanding slaveries that have occurred in the history of mankind. Millions of people today were never physically connected to either.

Legally, all these groups of slaves were set free thanks to abolitionists like William Wilberforce in the late 1700s to 1800s and Moses in the scriptures.

However, modern-day slavery is still practiced in over 160 countries[7] according to the U.S. State Department and affects 50–70 million people around the world. Slave mentality is still found in people all around the world from diverse languages, cultures, status, race, age, and gender.

Indecision

One major characteristic of slaves is that they are unable to withdraw from any arrangement. They live according to the dictates of their owners who make all the decisions on their behalf. This leads them to have a mentality of indecision. They can neither say yes nor no in a deciding moment. They are conditioned to know they have no say in any given matter.

This explains why to set the Israelites free from the slavery in Egypt God had to raise someone who though he was born into it didn't grow in the environment of captivity; a person who was raised in royalty; in the position of authority who had the ability to make decisions, someone who had a different mindset from the rest of the Israelites. Moses was this person God used to set his people free. The same is true for William Wilberforce. He was not of a slave descent but he used his position as a non-slave to advocate an end to slavery.

Trauma has buried the decisive abilities of many survivors. This is explainable if the events and people you once trusted placed you in the position where you were hurt and conditioned to be silent about it. It is understandable to move on, allowing anyone to say or do whatever they pleased without expressing an opinion, emotion or resistance.

Indecision is the greatest killer of achievement.

Today, so many have caged their greatness in the mindset of indecision. Many have been faced with life-changing opportunities, occasions to manifest their talents, events to showcase their abilities and locations to develop their gifts but because they are trapped in indecision, all these life-changing moments are left to pass away unutilized. Indecision is the greatest killer of achievement.

Lee Segal is associated with the saying, "A man with one watch knows what time it is. A man with two watches is never quite sure." I guess this was before the advent of technology because with the satellite now in place, all electronic devices seem to have the same time in the same location. Besides, very few people rely on watches to get information about the time. The watch has become more of just a piece of jewellery or another form of technology.

Anyway, the quote drives home the message. If you don't make the decision someone else will decide for you, and you may not be comfortable with the outcome. Your shepherd dwells within you. You must trust your one watch and not wait for a second watch to decide for you. This will only cause confusion to set in.

Don't mistake this to mean it is wrong to ask for advice. We should not mistake advice for indecision. Advice is meant to bring clarity while decision is acting on the clarification you got. Listen to your advisers, listen to yourself, then decide.

The advice from others should only give a broader perspective and breed more ideas. In the end, the ball is in your court whatever way you decide to play with it will determine the score you will get. Even the most valuable advice becomes useless if not used.

Strive never to be double minded because it will only lead to an unstable life. When instability sets in, failure is inevitable. It is often said the middle of the road is the most dangerous part of the road to be on. A car from either side of the road can run into you. We are made to be decisive in order to be productive.

EAGLE MENTALITY

Growing up, I learned about some very interesting creature: birds, animals, insects but the eagle was not one of them. In my elementary days and location, the eagle was not one of the popular creatures to teach the children. Moving on to preteens, I heard about the eagle a few times. From what I gathered from my little information it was an evil bird, which is very harmful and dangerous.

Later in life, reading through the scriptures and paying attention to the lyrics of some songs I heard in church, I discovered words like renewing the youth like the eagle and mounting on wings like eagles. Considering this information came from godly settings it baffled me as to why the good Lord would associate good things like strength, renewal with an evil creature like the eagle. This got me curious to find out more about the eagle. The results were so interesting that I decided to adopt the eagle mindset as revealed through its character. These characteristics make the eagle the head of the bird kingdom.

Renewal

Physically, an eagle goes through a renewal process to fly to higher heights, which symbolizes mental renewal a person should go through to move to the next level. When the eagle's feathers become weak and it cannot go the speed and height it anticipates flying, the eagle realizes that this inefficiency can lead to death. To avoid this avoidable circumstance, the eagle retires away to the high mountains.

Its purpose up in the mountains is to go through a very painful but much needed procedure of plucking out its weak feathers, beaks and claws from its body. It hits itself against a rock until its body is void of the feathers. After this, it stays in its hiding place until it grows new feathers, which will take it to new heights and new claws and beaks to allow it to be a better hunter.

At some point in life, we all need to come to the realization that our current mindset, habits, companions and acquaintances are preventing us from reaching higher heights. Many have a vision for their lives and know they can do more to become the person they desire but they keep holding on to the things that are weighing them down.

Quiet Time

Too many people operate in a victim, lack and slave mentality as opposed to the eagle mentality because they are too busy in their minds. Having a quiet time is out of place in many schedules though we all need and benefit from a quiet time for renewal like the eagle.

A busy mind can never achieve anything new because it is busy replaying what it already knows. It is accustomed to having a normal routine. A quiet time is a time to plan and schedule your day and life to gain more productivity. Have a quiet time to identify the roadblocks to recovery and pluck them out so you can fly higher.

A quiet time doesn't necessarily mean you have to go up a mountain or a remote area like the eagle. It is excellent if you have access to these resources but it is more of a mental procedure than a physical location. It is a state where the mind is relaxed and away from the distractions like technology. In quiet time, you intentionally tune off worry and physical contact.

Keep the mind in a liberal state so it can be filled with ideas and information that are needed for advancement. Sometimes the ideas and information you generate may not be for the immediate use and it may not look sensible, however write it down for sooner or later you will get the revelation for those words.

If you are like I used to be, you will say you don't have time to do this. Like everything else, it is a choice you should make and a priority to be on your schedule. If you are a morning person, I recommend you do this first thing in the morning if you have more energy at night, you can do this before going to bed, if you think you have more alone time during the day then schedule this at whatever time is more convenient for you. I once had someone ask me, what if I fall asleep in such a relaxed state. I told the person when you wake up, you can write in your journal: "I slept off." Whatever time of the day you choose, just do it for it will revolutionize your life.

Love the Storms

Another characteristic of the eagle worth copying is that it loves storms. Isn't that strange considering most of us dread both physical and emotional storms? An eagle uses the winds of the storm to lift itself higher and above the clouds. While the other birds seek refuge on the branches and leaves of trees during a storm while waiting for it to pass, the eagle uses the opportunity of the stormy winds to glide higher.

In life, we all face storms whether you hide from them or face them. Some interpret their storms as a season of stagnation or regression. Others, like the eagle, see them as an opportunity for acceleration. Be like the eagle and see your storms as a time of progression. When I took this stance, I could clearly see my stormy seasons as moments that push me steps further than I would have taken without a storm.

At the time of the storm, it seemed like nothing progressive was happening but as I practiced thanksgiving and bit my tongue several times not to complain and explain, when the storm was over, I realized I had been catapulted to a whole new realm of greater achievements. The stronger the storm, the higher it takes you somewhere you have never been before. Be grateful and be vigilant for the results.

Bury the Dead

The last characteristic of the eagle I want to point out is that unlike the vulture that feeds on dead things, the eagle feeds on fresh prey. The reason many people have not gone further up the ladder of recovery is because they held their minds captive in dead situations. Someone did something to you over twenty years ago, I bet you the person doesn't remember the event but you keep feeding on it, failing to see new opportunities to create new memories. Some of the events may not have been something unpleasant. It also applies to something great, sweet, successful worth celebrating. Whatever it was, celebrate it or mourn it, then let it go.

This doesn't imply that you forget the past but it is saying that you should use your past to learn principles to apply in the present and the future. Don't use your past to tell the old hag tale, which is beginning to sound like a broken record. Be willing to be filled daily with new experiences so your life will be renewed like the eagles.

> *Mental stagnation is devastating because it can be avoided.*

If you are wondering how did someone who was so bitter, negative, defeated, hopeless and faithless move from such a mindset to a victor and eagle mindset, I assure you it didn't happen in one day but it started one day, and it's a continual process of applying some basic steps on a regular basis, which I will share with you. It is a continual process.

STEPS TOWARDS A MIND SHIFT

The pace to a new mindset is what I call the AID process.

Acknowledge

Change is a choice, which can only be made when you realize that there is a need to change. Comfort in the present situation can never spark change. It can only come out of desperation or inspiration. It happens when you get to the point where you cannot let situations continue going in the same direction or you are inspired by the words of a writer, an artist, a picture, a teacher, coach or anyone you come across that speaks straight into your heart. In my case, I came to a point of desperation where I had to say enough is enough. I cannot continue to let circumstances control me, I want to take control of my life.

No one can force change on anyone. There is a saying that you can take a horse to a stream but you cannot force it to drink water. The people around you may see the unfavourable situation you are in, some may offer advice, others may give resources, but nothing will cause you to change until you acknowledge your need for it.

> It all begins with acknowledging that there is something that must change.

You must choose to have control over certain aspects of your life, choose the direction you want it to go. You have the power to choose what you allow in your life and what you kick out. That may not be the power you had earlier in life, but it is time to take it back. It all begins with acknowledging that there is something that must change.

George Bernard Shaw said, "Progress is impossible without change and those who cannot change their minds cannot change anything." If you are willing to change your mind you have taken the major progressive step. It might sound so simple and you're wondering if it happens just like that. The answer is yes! The greatest difficulty is to say yes! I have a limiting mindset and I am willing to let it go so I can become a better person.

The day you truly decide you don't want to feel and think in a certain way anymore is the day you change. Assess your current mindset and notice where it is leading you. If the destination is not favourable then it is time to take another route. I acknowledge that it takes a lot of courage to **let go of the familiar to embrace the fabulous** but it is worth it and you can do it.

> The real enemy is the enemy in the spirit, the enemy of the mind.

Identify

Congratulations, if you have taken the big step of acknowledging that some things need to change to get what you desire. The next step forward is to identify the enemy. U.S General Douglas McArthur said, "One of the most important rules of war is to know your enemy." This doesn't only apply to physical war but to the war in the mind as well.

The root cause of toxic mindsets of victim, lack and slave is fighting the wrong enemy. The word fight is not as bad as we think it is. What makes it bad is whom you fight physically. It is easier to be bitter when you fight against flesh and blood because they are not the real enemy. The real enemy is the enemy in the spirit, the enemy of the mind.

I harboured so much rage against my violators until I came to the realization that the people who violated me are just as ignorant as me. Of course, they thought they were smart and taking advantage of a vulnerable girl but they acted under the influence of a toxic spirit.

They had let the enemy plant bad ideas in their minds and were just living out the seeds they had grown.

When we realize the enemy is not the flesh and blood that hurt you, then you will take the battle to the right battlefield, which is the mind. I do not see myself as a victim anymore because I had to take the victory over the enemy from my mind. From that point, I stand in a position of victory, not a prey trying to get victory.

I ditched the lack mentality because I know I have all I need; I am just discovering them one at a time. I do not have the slave mentality anymore because I realized my mind has been set free, and I am endowed with the ability to make the right decisions.

The realization that this was a spiritual battle and my enemy had been defeated brought me total liberation. This caused me to change my mentality and adopt on purpose the victorious eagle's mentality, which brought me to a whole new level.

Decide

Socrates made a powerful statement when he said, "The secret of change is to focus all of your energy, not on fighting the old but on building the new." The new is built by getting knowledge of the new creation you want to become. It is logical that if you want to be smart study smart people, if you want to be wealthy study wealthy people, if you want to be successful, study successful people if you want to recover study those on a higher level on the ladder of recovery. You can also study the opposites of these people but just make sure you only learn what not to do. I recommend you focus your energy on the good stuff.

Knowledge breaks the depth of whatever has been buried deep within your heart and causes the clouds in your mind to drop down dewdrops of new information on any infertile situation. With knowledge, you can dig out revelations, which will cause things to begin to work in your favour. It is like dew just falling on you wherever you go. Some call it luck, I call it favor.

The best transforming knowledge you can ever get that will dramatically change your mind is the knowledge of who you are. For example can you imagine that out of the over 7.6 billion people on earth your creator loves you? That means if He has a smartphone you are under his contact list of favourites. Doesn't that make you feel special? In fact, I am blushing while I write this.

You could ask how do I know He loves you? I understand doubts may arise from all the things that have happened to you in the past and present but His Manual says so and His Words have been proven to be forever true. He loves you so much that he is letting you read this so you can reset your life.

It doesn't matter what everyone else thinks you are or how you consider yourself. It is just incredible that THE one who made the entire universe has a deep interest in you and loves you unconditionally. That revelation changed my life. It took me from low self-esteem to "high self-esteem."

Another great source of knowledge is motivational videos, books, and conferences. It baffles me how much time I used to spend reading news feeds, romance novels that mostly help ignite past hurts, violations, disappointments, and hate when that time could be spent getting knowledge what will guide me towards a brighter future or build a new foundation.

Winston Churchill said, "You will never reach your destination if you stop and throw stones at every dog that barks." Our world today is filled with so much information that pops up in your life often uninvited. If you pay attention to every information out there it will choke your destiny. You have to be intentional on what you allow into your mind. Stay focused on what you want and go after the knowledge that gets you there.

Your mind is more important than your body so why treat your body better than your mind? I am assuming you don't eat every food that is presented to you. You choose what to eat and what not to. We call some foods junk and others healthy. We cut out some foodstuffs from our diet to get a desired outward appearance and health goal; however, we absorb everything out there that takes us out of our mental goal and inward appearance.

I believe this is an invitation to a new season, and in order to get there you will have to break away from those things that are limiting your mind. That means you have to drop the garbage that is holding you back.

Choose wisely and don't be deceived. **Give up the wrong company but don't give up your life**. I understand from experience that the temptation to give up your dream is greatest when you are on the verge of getting something greater. Give up everything else but not your dreams.

JOURNEY WITH KIKI

After a deep reflection on this topic of mindsets, Kiki began to trace how her life had been influenced by her perception of herself.

"Following the death of my parents," she said, "I began to think I lacked everything I needed in life. It started with one thought: what if my parents were here? I would still be lavished with fancy gifts. Moreover, I wouldn't have to watch my father's relatives fight over our properties. Before I knew it, I was never contented with the basic needs handed down to me from my uncles and aunts. I complained about everything and had a desire to get something else to fill in for what I lacked.

When I made the wrong choices and didn't have the things I wanted, it pushed me deeper into the drain of defeat.

My earlier experiences shaped my mind into a mentality of defeat, failure, disappointment, and a victim. This doesn't mean that is always the reaction to occurrences like sexual abuse. Another person may have been sexually exploited, lost dear ones but had a different opinion of themselves. However I carried myself this way but I believe it is time to move forward, so I am willing to drop it to embrace a bright future."

REFLECTION

1. What are some mindsets that have dominated the course of your life?
2. What are some measures you can implement to step into a more fulfilling life?
3. Are there some habits you need to adopt or drop to embrace the new you?

CHAPTER 5:
RELEASE YOURSELF

Think twice before you speak, because your words and influence will plant the seed of either success or failure in the mind of another. —*Napoleon Hill*

At some point in life, we have had a person speak words to us that has defined our perception of ourselves. That is great if the words that defined your perception of yourself are words like, "You are great, you are successful, you are beautiful, you are creative, you have a bright future, you are a blessing ..." However, for most people, these are not the words they were told. What they heard sounded more like "You are a failure, you will never amount to anything meaningful in life, I regret the day I gave birth to you, don't bother trying because you will fail anyway, why can't you be like…"

The point is every single person on earth who has lived beyond five years of age has experienced these defining moments. It is defining because words are the most prevailing creative force in the universe. They bring disappointments, hardships, pain, and violations of personal expectations, joy, security, or mixed feelings.

Some of us were not sure how to receive and respond to those words so we just let them direct the course of our lives. However, if those words led you to a position you are not proud of, you have the chance to reverse the words you don't want and steer your life in the direction you want it to go. You could change all that by the words you speak or you could decide to continue carrying the weight of the hurtful words on your shoulders.

As you may have already experienced, the burden is not going to depreciate and get lighter because of the passing of time. Rather it will keep getting heavier because unless you become active regarding it, there will always be circumstances that will point out some truth in the words. Even minor details will be blown out of proportion.

TURN IT AROUND

You could choose to go around blaming everyone who verbally abused you for the unfavorable situation you are in but you have to face one truth: The mind that has harbored the words is a very powerful tool as we have seen in the previous chapter but something more powerful than the mind is the tongue; a representation of words.

Has someone ever asked you, what is your mother tongue? Or you may have heard the phrase, "They have a heavy tongue." That always relates to the spoken words. The mind is like the womb where the future is nurtured for a duration but words through the mouth is the channel that brings the future into the physical world. The future could be the next second or next twenty years from now, nevertheless, you will always get what you say.

Ideas and opportunities are conceived in the mind but they don't all see the world. You can have the most creative idea, the largest company the world will ever see, the cure for a deadly disease but if you don't speak it out there is a 99 percent chance that it will die a natural death and end up buried for good. The mind opens up potentials but only words bring them into existence. The choice is yours to turn the words around.

YOUR VOICE IS LOUDEST

If you are familiar with the scriptures you are likely familiar with how God created the world through words. If you are not familiar with the Bible, take a few seconds and open it to the first page of the first book of the Bible. It is written right there "and God said let there be … and there was …" you may say but that is the most powerful God, how can you compare me with Him? You are right; he is the most powerful God. He is a sovereign God but human beings also have their responsibilities. We are created in the image and likeness of God, which means whatever he did, he has given us the power to do the same through Christ, who said we shall do greater works than he did (John 14:12).

The challenge here is how do you use your words? We are to send our words in the direction we want our life to go because we can use our words to bring blessings or curses into our lives, we can use our words to bring life or death into any situation. I am convinced that if you are above twenty years, where you are today has a lot to do with the words you have been saying for at least the past five years.

On the other hand, if you are a person in authority over someone else; like a parent-child relationship, it could be that the outcome of your children has a great deal to do with the words you have been saying over them.

I once had someone ask me that what if there are two parents, one person is speaking good words while the other person speaks words which are not so good to the children, what is going to be the outcome? I know for certain that good overcomes evil. If you stick to the good, it will overshadow the evil. It may not happen in one day, it might take several years but it will definitely come to pass. The words you believe are the ones that will come to life.

You may never have intentionally cursed yourself or loved ones but you may have used some words you are accustomed to and it has led to an undesirable outcome. Several years ago, I was told an interesting life-changing story.

There was once a business woman who was a roadside vendor. She used to fry snacks on various sites and sell to passersby. One of the snacks she made is called puff-puff. On this fateful day, she was frying her puff-puff close to a football field, to sell to the fans and onlookers of the game. It wasn't a major sporting event, it was a local competition called "inter-quartier" between two neighbourhoods where kids came together to have fun playing football. Her son was one of the players in the game.

Every time she fried some puff-puff and put in a bowl to cool off, her son who was not actively playing would come over, take a handful and run off to wait for his turn to join the game. She scolded the boy a couple of times asking him not to come back for more, but he kept coming back. This made her upset as she was more concerned about the money she could make from selling those puff-puffs. She had valid reasons to be concerned, perhaps the sale would have yielded some of the much-needed money for her children's tuition, new clothes, shoes or a much-needed item.

Caught in her thoughts about her needs, her son came back for more puff-puff. As he took it and was about to leave she burst out in anger "chop die." This is a really common phrase in the environment where she lived. The phrase means to eat and die. Despite its significant meaning, it was taken as ordinary words, so some people smiled, others laughed, some didn't even notice what she said, and the woman certainly didn't wish to lose a son.

During his turn in the game, while the boy was playing he slipped and bumped his head severely on the goalpost. He passed on before he could receive any medical treatment. His mother believed prayers could restore her son's life so she started praying and pouring out her heart to God. She said while praying, she saw a scenario, which she shared later.

The woman recounted how an angel told her nothing can be done to bring her son back to life because she used her mouth to put an end to his life. Oh! What a tragic loss that could have been prevented if she had used life-giving words.

The results of words may not be as sudden and tragic as this story but they are inevitable. We often use our mouth to break things, break our lives or the lives of the people in our circle of influence but on the other hand we can also use our mouth to build our life and those of others. Just as words are used for creation, they can also be used for restoration in some cases. Recreation is the opportunity to build your lives again.

THE LAW OF SOWING AND REAPING

In part, where you are today is a result of the words you have been saying. Your words are seeds you are planting into your future. Imagine a farmer goes to a store and buys some grapefruit seeds. He gets back home, looks for a great spot and plants his seeds. Every day, first thing in the morning, he goes out to his grapefruit seeds and waters them. After watering the seeds, he sits on his couch hoping the grapefruit seeds will produce sweet, juicy oranges.

> **Most people plant seeds of death and expect to harvest fruits of life. It doesn't work that way.**

When harvest season comes he excitedly goes to his tree and expects to harvest his oranges. When he fails to harvest oranges, he feels disappointed and is bitter with everyone and everything around him. He blames the store attendant for selling the seeds to him. He blames the soil for not being fertile enough to produce the oranges, he blames the sun for not shining as much as the plant needed, he blames the rain and his watering can for not giving the plant enough water.

That is exactly how our lives have been designed. The Scripture says the tongue has the power of life and death and those who love it will eat its fruits (Proverbs 18:21). Most people plant seeds of death and expect to harvest fruits of life. It doesn't work that way.

You might say that is not me, I don't speak death I only talk about lack, defeat, disappointments, abuse, loss, hardships I am encountering, and the sicknesses in my body. My challenge to you is don't use your words to describe the situation you don't want to continue, rather use your words to paint the life of what you want to see.

You can say, I know I have been abused, violated, hurt, lost a dear one, valuable possessions but I am shaking off that event and rising to become the person who can be of service to me and to others. I may have failed at something but I am not a failure, I am rising to the realm of success. I might not have all I need to get what I want but good things are coming my way. I am entering a season of more than enough. When you speak like this, you are stirring your spirit to direct your life in the direction you want it to go. You are attracting the life you want to live and discarding what you have at the moment.

If you don't like the results of what you have been getting up to this point then it could be time for you to start planting a different seed. Don't look at problems, challenges and difficulties as things that have come to stay. Unless you invite them in, they remain passersby.

CURE TO CHALLENGES

> You are made to accommodate success and not problems.

When it comes to challenges, you should have the attitude of this too will pass because really you are made to accommodate success and not problems. That is why dwelling on challenges comes with stress and many stress-related sicknesses. That doesn't mean problems won't come. They will show up but when they do, you should know they are for a moment so rejoice because in joy, you will see a solution and blessings in the challenges.

Negative thoughts will always come during those trying moments but another challenge for you is to not speak them. Monitor your thoughts, identify the negative thoughts and don't give them life. You can simply tell it sorry you got the wrong address. I have changed my address from speaking killer words to speaking life-giving words so back to the sender. You can never defeat thoughts by thoughts so when the negative thoughts come up, defeat them by speaking out positive words. The victory lies in you hearing what you say. Don't cage your life in the trap of your words.

Most of the negative words we speak or accept as part of our lives are words people in authority over our lives may have said to you. People like your parents, guardians, teachers, ministers, politicians, friends, coaches, popular media, and social media. They will tell you what you can and cannot have. What you can and cannot do. Once we accept it that becomes our standard for life.

I have seen people who had been labelled with different words, which could cause them to get limited and live below their potential but when they came across a new truth that what was said to them is an individual's opinion and not the final say, these people have lived to achieve great things beyond their peers who were ranked in a higher category than them.

In my existence, I have realized that people who speak toxic words are mostly those who have had toxic experiences themselves. Why am I telling you this? So, you should not let what people say about you become the standard for your potential. The person may have gone through their own experiences and use that as a measuring rod for everyone else but because you are a masterpiece, only you can determine the limit you want to attain.

It is harder for children when words are used to define them and they can't speak back to correct the perception. I have heard parents use their own personal bias judgement to say words like "She is just shy." The child who doesn't even know what the word means grows up believing she is shy. She lives on to accept the label and live up to it. This could place a limitation on her ability to speak up when necessary.

On the other hand, I have seen parents who started saying their children are shy when someone tries to talk to them and they don't respond back. However, along the line, they discover that this could just be their opinion though the child acts in that manner. They correct this by telling the child words like, "You are not shy, you are bold, you are courageous, you are confident ..." I have seen these children rise to have a different personality and do things which they couldn't do before like becoming awesome public communicators. Don't let the opinion of people determine your destiny. There is nothing wrong with being shy, but I think there is nothing right with you living what you are really not.

In the case of children, they look up to people in authority over them to feed their young minds on the truths in this world but as we grow older we can remove certain labels placed over us or reject the words as soon as they are spoken. What we accept as children, whether right or wrong, shapes our lives. I have found myself acting on many false beliefs many years after I heard them spoken to me or overheard a conversation.

CURE TO NAYSAYERS

In certain parts of Africa like Nigeria and Cameroon, there is a sign people make when someone says a word to them which they don't agree should take hold in their lives. The person in denial lifts one or both hands and sways it over their head and say, "God forbid." What that means is, in the name of God, I forbid that word from coming to pass in my life, and I forbid it from staying on me. The thing is people have become so accustomed to the sign that they do it as often as they can but still live their lives under the influence of those words spoken over them.

What that tells me is that what matters is a reaction from the heart and not the action on the outside. Sometimes you may not be able to openly challenge the person in authority who says negative words to you but in your heart, you can press delete on those words and never dwell on them. You could one day bring it up as part of your testimony on how you rendered the words powerless and rose despite the challenge.

Some people have even intentionally dropped from being straight A students to a mediocre student because of the names from naysayers. Their friends gave them labels for always studying after school hours, called them "pompous" for asking questions to the teachers during classes, called them "showing off" for seeking clarification on a subject from the teacher after classes, called them "bookworm" for spending hours researching at the library.

To fit in and avoid those labels they intentionally stopped their quest for knowledge, they stopped the hobbies they loved and resulted with an average performance.

> *Remember! The pyramid of life is crowded at the bottom so every effort you make to get to the top will be accompanied by jarring and booing from those who have encountered hardship in certain areas of their lives in their own attempt to move up.*

Don't let a messed up person mess your life. Do yourself a favour to continue your journey so when you get to the top you can help them clean up their mess. You are blessed to be a blessing. Give a deaf ear to the name callers so you can make a name for yourself.

If your goal is to become the best version of yourself, then you must learn how to deal with the words people throw at you because they will always come. There is a saying associated with Eleanor Roosevelt that goes, "Great minds discuss ideas; average minds discuss events; small minds discuss people." It would have been better if small minds talk about you out of your hearing but the reality is they will talk in your presence or in a channel that will get to you. It is left on you to decide what to do with the words.

EXPECTATIONS PRECEDE WORDS

Your words are more powerful than the words of others. Use your own words to define your life.

You may want to reconstruct your life now but you have accepted the label given to you by others or you don't know in what direction to send your words.

You could start by setting your expectations for the outcome of your life. In our story of the farmer earlier in this chapter, our farmer had an expectation. He was expecting oranges though he planted grapefruit seeds so when you pick out your expectations, let it be what you really want to get.

What are you expecting? If you are in a difficult situation, you will have to be clear about your expectations for the future to speak the right words. For example, if you expect events to turn around in your favour, you can say I am blessed and highly favoured though you may not feel blessed or favoured. I once heard someone said, "Never let your feelings vote." If you expect the right ideas for the marketplace you could say, I am a great thinker and a great achiever. If you have an expectant heart and the right words, your problems will begin to see possibilities and you will take the right actions.

It is never too late to redefine your life. If you have breath you can still change the label placed on you by relabelling yourself. Your words are more powerful than the words of others. Use your own words to define your life. Never let the negative seeds of others grow in your heart because it will produce fruits that will be seen on the outside.

PERMISSION TO CONTROL

For too long you have given people permission to control your life. It is time to take back that permission and be the boss of your life. If you ever have to give someone control over your life why not give it to the one who knows you more than you know yourself, the one who created you and knows how best you are to function, the one whose voice you have silenced for so long because you are listening to people who don't even know who they are.

Why not give the control to God? The remarkable thing about God is that when you give your life over to Him, He makes you the co-pilot of the plane. That means He empowers you to become all that you want to be. The only limit is how far your expectations can take you.

When you accept the co-pilot seat God has offered you, take the Manual He has given you and find out all the great words He has for you. The Bible is full of so many unclaimed promises and blessings. However, because we don't take time to read it or our minds are so negative that we focus on the judgements and curses, we fail to see the glorious life we have been given. Give Him the chance to use you and do a makeover in your life.

ROADBLOCKS TO THE NEW YOU

Fear

One of the things that keep people from taking control over their life is fear. There is so much fear in the world that it has become normal to be fearful and abnormal when someone says I am not a slave to fear. Sometimes when you watch the news, read the papers or browse through social media fear grips you because of the things that fill the headlines. I once heard someone say, "Fear and worry are interest paid in advance on something you may never own." That is true but it also prevents you from getting something you may own.

Most of us love to sit on a deck with a beautiful view to watch the sunset or a beautiful display of light and absorb the accurate view. When it comes to the circumstances of our lives, the most accurate view of your future is not from a position of fear but from a position of faith. Fear will only bring in failure, disappointments, heartbreaks, frustration, and a pool of tears. Above all, fear has stopped many people from following their dreams.

In order to defeat fear, you must have faith and exercise your faith. Fear comes to the mind of everyone but those who choose to live by faith do not exercise their fears but rather respond to situations by faith. Fear believes that you will not get the things you desire to have, faith on the other hand, believes you are qualified to have the things you hope to get though it is not in your hands right now, it is coming because your faith is the evidence you need. When you receive something in the spirit nothing can stop it in the physical so be careful where you put your hope.

Therefore, it is a choice for you to have the good things in life that you desire. You can change the circumstances that concern you but most definitely, not by just sitting head bowed down and hoping that nothing bad happens to you.

You have to decide how to make use of the skills, talents and abilities you have in you. Don't be worried that you may not be so good at the things you want to do when you first do them, it often takes more practice to get better at it. All you should do is put in all your interest in it. Not part of it but all. Be fully present in what you do.

The word interest is an interesting one. It means attention but interest also means an additional charge on an initial deposit. What that tells me is that I have put in an initial effort then, and withcontinuity more return will come out of it. So therefore, you will have to put yourself out there as an initial deposit and become actively involved in what you want to get out of life.

Excuses

Another stop sign on the road to taking control of your life is excuses. I once heard the story of a lady who planned to go to college after her kids were old enough to be independent. It so happened that at the age of nineteen, her last child decided to leave home to stay in the university campus where she will be studying. This lady told her friend, you know it has always been my dream to go to college when the children leave home but a college degree takes four years.

I am forty-four years old now by the end of four years I will be forty-eight. I feel like I am too old to go to college. Her friend asked her, "If you don't go to college now, how old are you going to be four years from today." Shocked that she had to state the obvious, the lady said, "Hmmm … I will be forty-eight years old." Her friend said, "Yes, you are still going to be forty-eight without a college degree and wishing you had gone to college."

Sometimes the excuses we give for taking control of our lives are genuine, like not having the right connections, the lack of finances, too young or too old. However, whether we take control and do what we want to do or not, those hindrances will always be there. All we need to do is to change our focus.

You should do whatever you need to do that will give you a sense of fulfillment. It will be different from person to person so you will have to focus on your own fulfillment not the fulfillment of others. You will face opposition, you will face challenges but if you are on your side you don't need anyone else to be there with you. If you have the support of friends and family that is a plus – not so many people have that. If you don't, it's nothing to worry about. On the journey to being yourself many of your current passengers will drop along the road, you just keep going till you get there. I hope this information you get leads to action not just knowledge.

Negativity

Before the advent of digital cameras and smartphones there were single-lens reflex (SLR) cameras that produced negatives. When you look at the negatives of the pictures, you had to guess which ones you wanted to print because the negative was blurry. You couldn't tell the exact details of the image; the position of clothes and jewellery; if there was an unwanted shift, the posture, and the facial expression. The negatives don't give the exact picture you want but when they are developed and printed, you see all the details you had missed in the negative. That is exactly how our lives work. If you focus on the negative you miss the beautiful picture that will be produced but if you wash out the negative you will see a beautiful print of the situation or your future life.

FOR INSPIRATION NOT PITY

Have you ever called someone on the phone, as soon as the person picks up the call the first sentence is "What happened?" and you are like "Hmmm ...? Nothing happened! I just called to ..." and the next thing you hear is "What are you hiding from me? Is everything okay?" Often by the end of that call you are like "What just happened to me?" Some people are so focused on getting negative news that they only expect to hear bad news. If you tell them something positive they think you are acting nice or sweet coating something bad. If you're not careful they suck the energy out of you.

Focus your energy on the positive. What you listen to has a great impact on you, what you remember has a greater impact on the outcome of your life. There are negative things in everyone's past. Are you going to draw strength or pain from your past?

It is so easy to go through life with baggage that is weighing us down, let's face it, after all you have been through being negative is the natural thing to do. But the thing is, beneath the negative are the positive and joy-filled moments. It is often easier to talk about the bad things that happened to us than the good memories unless we make it a priority to focus on good memories.

Take control of how you reflect and talk about the issues of your life. My father passed away when I was eight years old. For the longest time, I lived in denial that his death had any effect on me. In secondary and high school, every time a friend lost a parent and I saw their anguish, I would say to myself, it's a good thing my father died when I was eight years old and at a time when I had few memories of him. I will move on to remind myself of the things I would have done better if he was still alive. All that did was bring tears and pain pushing me deeper into grief.

When I started focusing on the fond memories I had of him, the ones filled with joy, laughter and happiness, they always brought a smile to my face. Whenever I have thoughts of my father dying, the incident of his last days playing in my mind, I would switch that with the good memories I have of him. Dwelling on the good memories will not bring him back to life but it will renew my strength to face life with positivity.

> You can have a whole new life in front if you decide to drop the past and face the future.

You should consider letting go of the stories of the people who offended you and offend you. If you are on planet Earth people will continue to offend you. You may choose to dwell on it or delete the incident and focus on the good stories or some other exciting incident. I understand it could be hard to have fond stories of someone who abused you but if you are in a safe environment now, talk about those incidents for inspiration and not for pity. If you had such experiences, what have you achieved being bitter and resentful? You have to empower yourself by dropping the hurt and move forward in your life. Don't imprison your destiny because someone hurt you. They may be living their life while you are in a cage mourning about how they didn't treat you right. Your past is not supposed to determine your future, you can have a whole new life in front of you decide to drop the past and face the future.

Often, the emotional hurts are more dangerous and painful than the physical hurt. The people who hurt you sometimes forget they had done something wrong to you but every time you remember it and dwell on the tiny details of the incident, you give the person the power to keep hurting you. Unless you empty out the bad memories you cannot make room to let good words flow out of you because even if the good things come, you will face them with a negative attitude and so miss the blessing in it.

When you focus on the negative things, not only do they prevent you from enjoying everyday life, they also eat up the best in your future. If you decide not to dwell on the negative words, you will realize that it takes less energy to focus on speaking good words than you imagined.

Not only does it take your energy, but it also takes so much time to invite the things you do not even want in your life. If you save that energy and time, the reward will blow your mind when you break the piggy bank of your energy/time deposit. You will realize that your productivity has increased in ways you could never imagine.

Stop putting up a pity party and having that "hear what I have been through attitude" because majority of the people you invite to the party don't care. The more your conversations with people dwell on your hurt from a position of pity and who didn't treat you right, the more you push them out of your life. On the other hand, if you keep telling people your story for inspiration, the good reports, you attract them to you because hey who doesn't like good reports? Believe it or not, everyone wants to be surrounded by positive people, even the toxic people you know are looking for positive energy to neutralize them. Share your story for inspiration not for pity.

Turn that pity party into a burial ceremony. Get a casket, put in the bad words, have a funeral and bury it. Just like you never want to dig up a corpse that has been buried for days, months and years, never attempt to dig up that negative memory because you won't want to stand the stench that will come up with it.

JOURNEY WITH KIKI

After days of reflection, Kiki could see clearly how her words had influenced the present situation in her life. When she fell in love and married her husband she always said it was too good to be true because she just didn't see how her marriage was going to last. Her past experience of loss landed her in the belief that she would not have a long-term relationship.

All through her courtship and early years in her marriage to a man who she describes as a dream come true; a man who has all the good qualities she hoped for. Yet she kept saying she is unworthy of such a relationship so it is going to come to an end soon. At the time, there was nothing to warrant such confessions but because she held on to the belief, those good qualities began to turn sour.

It took this new revelation for her to realize that she may have invited her current situation into her life. With a recognition of her role in the crisis, she began to plan on how to make things right. Part of her plan was to stop speaking death into the dying relationship if she wants it to live again.

CHAPTER 6:
WHAT IS YOUR WORTH?

Self-Esteem comes by being able to define the world in your own terms and refusing to abide by the judgment of others. —*Oprah Winfrey*

We have all had things happen to us which makes us question our value; if we are worth being loved, worthy of respect, worthy of friendship, relationships and life itself. No matter what happened to you, know this: you are priceless, you are an irreplaceable treasure, and you are worth much more than you can imagine.

Do not let the words of the human traffickers make you believe that you are worth a few dollars. Do not base your value on the goods, services and money that was exchanged with those who sexually exploited you. All they did was to try to bring down your value. Don't give them the joy of believing they succeeded. Rise up and take your place as the most precious person who ever existed. No one is more valuable to you that you are. Determine your worth!

Your value comes from what you have in you not outside of you. It comes from your gifts, talents, your love and your smile. The good news is that we all have this deposited in us. More so, as long as you have breath, there is someone somewhere waiting for something: it's in you to make their life better. That is how valuable, highly esteemed and worthy you are.

Everyone you meet walking down the street has experienced their share of hurts. Their story may not be exactly like yours but I guarantee you, there is someone going through what you have gone through. The best you can do for yourself at this moment is to take your mind off yourself for a minute, go out there and help someone out there who is hurting.

Use your words, your smile or whatever you have to make yourself more valuable. Don't give the pain a chance to fasten-in your potential.

SELF-ESTEEM CONS

Low self-esteem arises from what I call the Triple A's of Esteem.

Abusers

Abusers are those people who use their position to treat others cruelly. It could be someone in a close relationship like – a parent, child, partner, spouse, sibling or relatives. It could also be a neighbour, friend, acquaintance, anyone in authority or someone you meet for the first time and may never have contact with again.

While all forms of abuse like physical (violence and neglect) and sexual abuse, I find emotional abuse more grievous because it is often present in the various forms of abuse. It also sometimes occurs independently and it is often unrecognized yet its repercussions are always present.

> How you esteem yourself should not come from how another person treats you. You are so valuable that you should not give another person the power to control your worth.

Emotional abuse is mainly responsible for blanketing a person's confidence and self-esteem. We often recognize it verbally through the harsh, negative and insulting words others pour on us but how about the non-verbal cues we often miss to recognize like manipulation, isolation, control, withholding, belittling and threatening. These also dampen self-esteem.

How you esteem yourself should not come from how another person treats you. You are so valuable that you should not give another person the power to control your worth. It doesn't matter what you have heard concerning your conception, birth and nurturing, one thing that is certain is that an unwavering value was deposited into you at the time you were created. It is time to recreate yourself by taking back the power you may have unconsciously given to your abusers.

Whether you were raised by your biological, adopted foster parents or extended relatives, know that you were so valuable at creation that you were worth loving and keeping so you could see the world. So many people walking down the streets have lost that initial value placed on them to experiences, circumstances and opinions of others.

The disheartening treatment from a few people in my lives made me devalue myself. Yes, now I can say there are a few people because if I look back at my life while growing up, I came across several friends, well-wishers, teachers and family members who treasured me and some went above and beyond to take care of me and nurture me but then I was wallowing in self-pity and failed to recognize their efforts. It is time to drop the schemes of the abusers and wear the crown of your true identity.

You can sit back and wallow in the lies your abusers made you believe or you can rise up and take control over your God-given potential. The choice is yours to make. As for me, I choose to say, "I am in control here, I will not allow anyone to determine my feelings and value."

Actions
You are Not What You Did
Sometimes too, we devalue ourselves based on the things we have done or items we are addicted to. What you did is different from who you are. What you find yourself doing no matter how hard you are trying to disconnect from it does not determine who you are. What you struggle with is different from who you are. You may have failed at

something but that doesn't make you a failure. Your value is far greater than your performance.

The fact that you had sex before and outside marriage doesn't make you a prostitute. The fact that you stole something doesn't make you a thief. Take off the label you placed upon yourself which is making you act in accordance to the label. So many people made a mistake once but because they felt that their value is measured by that mistake, they choose to continue with that act because they think it already defines them. That is a lie the enemy of your soul wants you to believe.

The best step to take is to confess that act to anyone in authority over you or a trustworthy person in your life. You don't have to confess because you just want someone to know about it. The reason you confess is because you want to take the burden of the action away from your mind so it stops tearing you apart within. Confession could also help you find the support you need to stay away from that act.

Among the many actions that made me feel worthless and suffering low self-esteem for most of my teenage years and into my adult life, binge eating is one act that stands out the most. This is because I knew there was a word for my action but I didn't know what it was. Even as an educated young adult, I had never heard the words. If someone had said it in my hearing, it didn't matter much to me so it failed to register in my brain. I was perishing in my lack of knowledge on that subject.

Although I knew there was something wrong in this eating habit because it brought in feelings of guilt and low self-esteem, I didn't know how to help myself. I remember a few friends during my university days that used to make mockery of how much food I consumed but that didn't help me in any way except to plunge me deeper into the pit of low self-esteem.

Perchance if I knew what it was; if I knew this was my maladaptive method of coping with my flashbacks of trauma I could have been liberated from it much sooner. However, I believe everything happens at the right time. You are smart, wise and intelligent but knowledge is broad and constantly growing just like you so you need the help of others to grow in the knowledge of the area where you need help.

It is easy to have low self-esteem if you base your worth on what you have done, what accusations have been placed on you, how they treat you and worse still what you think the people in your life are saying about your actions.

Do not let the mistakes you have made determine who you are and keep you in the circle of those mistakes. You can turn your life around into the future you desire and you deserve. You are greater, stronger, smarter, wiser and higher than you think. Give yourself another chance to re-evaluate yourself from the standpoint of your internal values and not your actions.

Accomplishment

The most insecure place a person can be is at the place of zero self-worth and not zero net worth. Sadly, that is where most of us are left after abuse and trauma. Some people have gone ahead to achieve great net worth despite the challenges they faced earlier in their lives yet they still have a zero balance in their self-worth.

Many of us lived with the battle of viewing ourselves as a valuable person although our bosses may appraise the job we do, friends and family members are proud of what we have acquired while everyone else sees the value in us, we find it hard to pick out those things they see. If that sounds like you, don't torment yourself about it because the truth is that our accomplishments are not a replica of our true value. Net worth is never equal to self-worth.

This problem of not seeing our value always arises from basing our value on external factors. What do you see outside of you: cars, houses, jobs, money, parenting, award-winning spouse … what do they see outside of me? To hide the inner struggle, many turn to what possessions they can acquire to have a good praise report from onlookers as oppose to the criticism we perceived though the words are not verbalized.

There is nothing wrong in having all possessions and connections, they could increase your influence but don't let it be a base for your value because if you do get those things and feel valuable then you are likely to lose your life or have a devastating crash if something goes wrong with all the things that determine your value.

Most of us were raised to associate value with money and properties but never did I imagine that it could be associated with who you are without those things. However, I later came to realize that if you determine your personal value without the external possessions, you will be able to determine how much money and properties are accorded to you.

What I mean is, look inward into your capabilities, your talents, your gifts, the minute things we seem to bypass; our smile, genuinely offering a helping hand to someone in need, listening to the hurt of a weary person, giving a word of encouragement to the broken-hearted, celebrating with the victorious and being genuinely present in our relationships. These are some of the things that showcase our true value and increase our self-esteem.

> If you can't say something to someone at least to their face then don't say it to yourself.

Besides the material possessions, one accomplishment that causes devastation to set in is body image. In my case being a mother at fifteen and my maladaptive coping mechanism of food made me suffer from a severe form of negative body image. After overeating and looking at my body, out of shame and disappointment in myself, I will resort to describing myself in ways I would never consider describing another person. My word to you is that if you can't say something to someone at least to their face then don't say it to yourself.

This negative image caused me to always feel unattractive. However, when I look back at my pictures from those days, I marvel at how physically good looking I was. I wish I could have seen myself from that perspective at that time but I don't regret my distorted view because I learned some valuable lessons for that experience I would like to share with you.

- Recognize that you did not develop your body image all on your own. The people in your life and society (culture and media) influenced it. When you recognize this, you will realize that you cannot fit into the mould of everyone so put yourself first and be who you want to be.

- Natural processes like childbirth and ageing change your body. It is okay if you don't get back to who you were physically before the process. Love what you have now while you hope and work on growth in the areas you want to grow. Be grateful for what you received and the lessons you have achieved through the process.
- Emotions change our body image so if you feel negative about your body, switch your thoughts to something that gives you positive energy. Something that makes you feel happy, loved and grateful.
- Tell yourself what you will tell someone you love who comes to you complaining about their body.
- The people you are trying so hard to fit into their mould may not even see the flaws you see in yourself.
- Keep in mind that you owe it to yourself to love your body as it is because it is the house that accommodates all you need to become. You cannot hate your way into loving yourself.

SIGNS OF LOW SELF-WORTH

Criticism: sensitive to criticism or being too critical of others.

> If you ever need something for comparison, compare your present state to your past in measurement of your future.

Are you the kind of person who is sensitive to criticism? If you are, don't hesitate because I understand where you are coming from. Most trauma survivors had been put there by people they looked up to for encouragement and affirmation. It is no wonder that at a certain point later in life they turn out to be sensitive to critics when they put in their utmost best in a task. We all know criticism can be coming from a constructive or a destructive standpoint. However, if you are someone who gets worked up without looking into the criticism to examine if there is some truth in it, then it is time to check how you view yourself.

It could be you are still look up to the praises of people to feel good about yourself so when you get criticized instead of praised, you esteem yourself from that person's judgement. That should not be the case. You are a priceless treasure irrespective of whether someone is trying to make you better or just trying to put you down.

Also, do not be overly critical of yourself. I know it is not as easy as it sounds, especially when your life stands out from your peers though not in an awesome way. When your life stands out as that kid in the neighbourhood everyone points fingers at and whisper when you passed by, I won't tell you it is easy not to condemn yourself but what I do know is that self-condemnation will lead to devastation and ruin your life if you don't lay it down.

On the flip side of this is that you could be the one being too critical of others. This might be a surprise to you but it is also a sign of low self-esteem. Do not criticize others simply because there is something in them, something they did which is triggering to you so you just have to say something about them though your observation will not build them. Any words you say which are not out to build, encourage, teach or help others grow are words you will probably regret in the future.

Do not judge or criticize others simply because you just want them to know your opinion on their plans and accomplishments. That could be a sign that you either are consciously or unconsciously measuring your value with them. If you ever need something for comparison, compare your present state to your past in measurement of your future.

Thinking poorly about yourself

The general thoughts you have about yourself will reveal how you esteem yourself. If you think you are a failure, a disappointment and will never accomplish anything good. Guess what? You will never value yourself above your thoughts. It is time to turn around those negative thoughts by giving yourself a pep talk.

This is an area I struggled with for years until I did what I am asking you to do now. You could use a pep talk to help you drop that condemnation. My first pep talk was a phrase I picked up from the Bible. It is a scripture which says, "There is no condemnation for those who are in Christ Jesus." (Romans 8:1). I knew my position in my relationship with God but I found myself in a position where I had lots of doubts if I was eternally condemned or if I could ever rise up and live guilt free from my past, which affected my self-image.

I had to pep talk myself to believe that again. I repeated those words again and again until I realized I was no longer my favourite critic. There are already a lot of people out there against you and there will always be, so do yourself a favour and be on your side and not on the opposition. Find the words that light up your spirit and give you hope. Speak them repeatedly until you come to believe them. As time goes on, build up your repertoire of pep talks in every area of your life. You will not regret that you did.

Body language
Another sign of feeling worthless is the way you carry yourself around; non-verbal communication. In the past, if I finally happened to leave the house after staring at myself in the mirror, I would go out with a head bowed down carrying a heavy crown of shame. My signature posture was folded arms whether when walking, standing or sitting like it added some sort of confidence.

Body communication is not one of my skills but one thing I know for sure is when you move around with your head down and a defensive folded hand, you are communicating a message of a defeated victim, making yourself an object of interest for the devourer. I guess dear David in scriptures experienced this first hand, which is why he said, "But you, Lord, are a shield around me, my glory, the One who lifts my head high." Psalm 3:3.

All hope is not lost if you are still carrying yourself around with that posture. The Lord who acts as a shield around David and lifted up his head is still available and more than willing to do the same for all who call upon Him. Give Him a call and enjoy the benefits of His response.

While you are at it, practice looking at yourself eyeball to eyeball in the mirror so you can be more confident to look others in the face when talking to them as opposed to avoiding eye contact as was customary for me. I could give up an opportunity to have an in-person conversation. Emails and mobile phones helped to ease my problem but some situations are better handled in person than through communication devices. You don't want to miss that dream job because your physical contact transfers a message of insignificance or lack of confidence.

Inflated status and possessions
Many people go around over representing themselves in order to match up with the status others will regard as worthy. This is a sign of low self-esteem to look out for. There is nothing wrong with having big dreams if it gets you to where you want to be. However, it becomes defective when you want people to see you in a certain way because in your opinion those with such possessions and status are more valuable than you are. Thus portraying that is a way to make you feel good about yourself without taking into consideration if there is a repercussion when your true self is revealed.

Another side of this is being a people pleaser. This implies you will do anything for anyone who has something you admire because you believe they are better than you. I am of the opinion that it is very rewarding to be of service to others but that should come from a place of love and not low self-esteem.

It will be evident that a service is not provided out of love when you either compromise your values to make others happy or you withhold your honest opinion because you don't want the other party to get offended by your response.

There have been many occasions in my past that I feel bad that I didn't contribute during a decision making process when faced with an opportunity to do so. In those times I would just say, "Do what you want." To be honest, I thought I was just an easygoing person so I didn't want to bring in complications if I said something contrary, but the truth is that I valued the opinions of others more than mine. So I kept my contributions to myself because I esteemed them to be very insignificant though vital.

Now I know better. I know I was saying I am not valuable, my words and action don't count so do whatever you want, you are better than me. Even without saying these words, in the long run, the people you often deal with will stop consulting your opinion. At that time, you would have indeed lost your value for contribution to them. That is the point to which I got. If you are not there yet, you don't have to get there. Start by saying as few words as possible until you are more confident to describe your entire view.

Rejects Compliments

Also, if you are like I used to be, that is never accepting compliments, it is a sign that you don't value yourself and don't see why you should believe those who see value in you to the extent that they give you compliments. In your opinion, you think they are sugar coating your errors so instead of accepting the compliments you turn it around and make them feel bad for offering those sweet words.

Dear friend I know this could be hard but when next someone makes the effort to complement your dressing, your work or something nice they see in you, take a deep breath and say, "Thank you." These two words will bring so much relief. It will help you digest thoughts, purge the negative thought and not voice it out. It will also make you think twice about the compliment. Maybe they could be right. Maybe there is something nice in you after all and if you dig deep, you will see there is indeed lots of good stuff about you.

Abusive or Tolerating Abuse

You may have heard the saying that those who are hurt tend to hurt others, while that is true, it is also true that those who have been hurt tend to accommodate more hurts. In the first case, those who have experienced hurt may turn out to be very hypersensitive to information and expressions so may tend to react aggressively towards others physically or verbally because they have the tendency to be defensive in order to avoid perceived upcoming abuse.

This could also be a response from the nervous system to a trigger as explained by the neurobiology of trauma and may require intervention from a practitioner in that field. However, it could also be an indication of low self-esteem if your reaction is because you interpret the intention of the other person as an attempt to belittle you. Make a choice to be confident in yourself so that the actions and words of others will not put you down.

On the other hand, most people who have experienced trauma tend to accommodate more traumatic experiences either because they have been accustomed to them and do not see a way out of the situation or you just think they can never be treated better so why not just make do with what they have. Inasmuch as that could be comforting to you, you should never settle for less than you deserve.

You deserve the better treatment and life you desire and you can have it if you refuse to settle with the hurt you are experiencing. I may not know the exact solution to get you out of the situation you are in right now, but if you change your mind from a worthless consciousness to you being valuable, you will see a solution that will make you get want you want.

Blaming

Are you still living in the story of the source of your abuse? I respect your story but in order for you to move on you will have to stop telling the story as the victim. Which implies you should stop blaming the people who abused you. This doesn't mean they did not do something wrong to you, it simply means you are more valuable than their maltreatment. Your self-worth should not be measured by their treatment; however, that is exactly what you are saying each time you say "do you know what … did to me?

They may not have known your worth, they may have tried to destroy your value if they had an idea of it but don't give them the chance to think they have succeeded by you feeling low about yourself. Do not blame them and do not blame yourself either. Yes, the experience was painful, there are no words to justify it but drop the blame and pick up your crown. There is a silver lining in that cloud, search for it and dwell it on instead of the blame. The silver lining might just be the fact that you are alive. Blaming will make you dwell on their actions and miss your value. You are so valuable to be here today.

REVALUE YOURSELF

True self-worth, value, esteem or whatever you choose to call it all comes from one source: the one who made you. You are a masterpiece; there is no one on this earth exactly like you irrespective of if you are an identical twin or a clone. One more thing, when God created me and you, He said this is "very good" Genesis 1:31. That means anything that tells you otherwise is not from the creator so it should not be part of you.

Don't let abuse, actions and accomplishment tell you otherwise. Those things don't determine your value, God does and to Him, you are very good. You can go on a diet, exercise, enrol in a course, get a better job, buy a new car, move to a better house, create new contacts; those things don't make you more valuable because you are already as valuable as you can be. They will only help you develop your talents and gifts, achieve your goals and accomplish your purpose, increase your net worth but it has nothing to do with your self-worth.

The true self is in the heart not the person on the outside so start working on your value from the inside and soon it will be evident on the outside. Change your focus from your external features to your internal features, and slowly but surely, you will start seeing your esteem changing.

You are very valuable to yourself, your family, the community and the world whether they know it or not so esteem yourself in high regard because there is no one exactly like you. People may look like you, talk like you, walk like you, smile like you, cry like you, do task and jobs like you but no one else can do it exactly like you. There is something special about you, which only you possess. That makes you very worthy.

You were made for good things to happen to you so don't stoop low to mediocrity because you think you are not worthy of getting a better deal. If there is one person in your life that deserves to be happy that would be you. You can only give out what you have so you must be happy to give out happiness to the people you love and care about.

JOURNEY WITH KIKI

Kiki's view of herself had been altered by all three cons of self-esteem. At a point, she viewed herself with great esteem because she was given all the things she desired as opposed to some of her childhood peers who lacked some of the basic necessities of life.

As time went on, she developed a mixed perception when her father started abusing her sexually. Being so young, she felted valuable because her parents constantly showered her with gifts but on the other hand, her mother had blamed her for being the cause of her father's action. This weighed heavily on her esteem so at this point her view of herself fluctuated. Was she valuable or was she a problematic child?

Her husband's abusive behaviour later in the marriage, coupled with her belief that she will only be held in high regard by her relatives and community of friends based on how well she fits into their ideology of marriage, raising children and holding on to traditional values, shattered the little regard she had of herself. This made her ignore her personal values, vision and aspirations.

Although she became increasingly unhappy trying to meet their standards, to her living her life the way she desired was not an option because she had to be who they want her to be against all odds.

With the new knowledge she obtained came the realization that she had to start a search of herself. It dawned on her that she had somehow lost knowledge of who she truly is without what she received from others and how she was accessed by society. It was time for a search of who she is void of abuse, actions and accomplishments.

This search led her to discover that all along she had been striving to become something she already is but just didn't recognize. She was striving for things like love and acceptance. These are things she already had but didn't know because her search for this was in the wrong places.

When she discovered the truth of who she is, she began a practice of constantly affirming her identity. A constant practice of affirmation erases the lies, which caused higher self-esteem to set in and led her to the things she had always wanted.

Picking up her identity directed her to her destiny, the purpose of her existence, the things she could do beyond the limitations which had been on her. First, she had to change her view of herself in order to step into the worth attached to her.

CHAPTER 7:
CRAVING TO BELONG

To be yourself in a world that is constantly trying to make you something else is the greatest accomplishment. —Ralph Waldo Emerson

Life is full of relationships; it is almost inevitable not to be in one form of relationship at any given time in your life. Every second you look around, you find yourself in a relationship with someone else. It could be with a neighbour, a partner, a friend, a boss, a pet, someone on social media you don't know personally and may never get to meet in person, a person you meet on the street. We are in a constant circle of interactions.

For some people, these interactions can take place with ease, but for most of us who have experienced one kind of trauma or another, it is a struggle getting into, building, and maintaining relationships. Many have experienced a breakdown of trust in themselves and the world, which has shielded the possibility of a satisfying relationship. Others had the capacity of a healthy relationship stripped from them even before they could correctly pronounce their name.

Irrespective of the process that brought about the challenge of a healthy relationship we still crave for a healthy relationship; to be part of a union or a community though there is that barrier or fear to engage in it. That fear has caused some to resort to solitude though that craving still lingers.

We all have different stories when it comes to engaging in intimate relationships but they all boil down to 'I have tried before but it didn't work'; 'I tried, it seemed to be working so I invested my hopes and trust into it but it was dashed'; 'I have seen many people get hurt so I don't want to take the risk of putting myself in the position to be hurt.'

I hear you and I understand the place you are coming from. I have been on that journey and I can genuinely say it is not an easy road to travel. Most of the reasons we give for the relational challenges are formed by the opinions and actions of other people.

EARLIER THAN YOU IMAGINED

Breaking free from those opinions is not always easy because as humans we are made to belong, to connect and to rely on others. This starts right after conception. We had to rely on our mother for nutrients during the period of gestation. It continues even after birth without the use of spoken words. When a baby cries, they need someone to pick them up and cuddle them, tell them it is okay; I am here for you, you belong to me now, I will take care of you and your needs. Some never had this experience and this is the commencement of relational challenges.

As the baby grows to a toddler and young kids, they need constant affirmation from their caregivers that they care about them; they will protect them. When children get this they tend to trust those caregivers as their safety spot.

At the point when this is broken, children at any stage even at teenage years will look for a place to fit in because they need that sense of belonging. For most people who have encountered abuse, violations and exploitation as children, they often grow up with that imprint of betrayed trust and lack of belonging. Some of us still had that physical belonging to our families, friends and peers but emotionally we belong nowhere.

Emotionally, we have that pain we do not talk about but we act out. As a mother, I often tell my children to use their words when they seem to act out their needs. But do you know most of us as teenagers and adults still act out our need for belonging? We act it out by numbing it with substances, cutting ourselves, attacking others verbally and through actions, seeking connections on the Internet; which often leads to using sex as a currency, exploitation, or we act it out by staying silent.

Diasporic trauma is one area where the need for belonging is often displayed though overlooked. As a migrant in another country, I find many people from similar backgrounds making poor choices because they want to feel accepted in a new community, they want new friends to make up for the ones they have left behind in their home countries.

Many of these immigrants have suffered various forms of trauma and abuse, which are unresolved but have been treated by a culture of certainty. A culture that tells them you react to your pain by shutting up and forget the incident ever happened. Did that make the pain go away? No! Did that create the sense of belonging we long for? No!

I once adopted that silent treatment perfectly. I packaged my pain and hid it securely deep within my heart while I went out searching for where I could belong, seeking to belong to a group of students who appeared happy and confident. In my thoughts, perhaps if I was part of that group I would have their happiness and confidence. Did that fill the gap? My answer is, no!

THE REWARD OF BELONGING NO PLACE

Joy in life comes when we make a choice to be content in every season of life. Though we crave relationships, there are moments when we find we do not belong anywhere else except to ourselves.

Most of the information we acquire has taught us that not being part of a group, part of someone's life is something worth weeping about but is that entirely true? As caregivers, educators, influential people in society teaching the younger generation and those of us adults who missed this lesson that there is blessedness in belonging no place will solve lots of societal problems.

From my experience, I am so grateful for the times I spent lamenting that I belonged nowhere. At that time, I faced my aloneness as cowardly isolation, where I would sit in my room and often cry myself to sleep, dreaming that I may end up alone for the rest of my life; thinking no one is ever going to accept me; I am not worthy of love and acceptance from any human being.

You find yourself

In a season of being alone, a time when some could say I was lonely and others would say I was living in isolation I learned to be my true self. I discovered the things I am passionate about and the things that turn me off. During that season, I learned the most valuable lessons: the real you is what you do in secret and, secondly, loneliness doesn't mean you are alone.

In my moments of reasoning when I was not lamenting, the books I read, the movies I watched and the places I went to when I dared to leave the house revealed to me my areas of interest. It is easy to lose our personal interest when we are trying to fit into a crowd. I used to hear a saying that two is company but three is a crowd, however even in a company of two you can lose your passion if the boundaries are not well defined. Unless you love your lone self, you cannot love you in the company of others.

Power of quiet time

Another lesson I learned is the power of quiet time. If you ever find yourself alone make it a habit to practice having a quiet time; a time to relax the mind and receive revelations to unanswered questions and direction to the desired destination. If you have ever been silenced about a situation, I bet if you had practiced a time of silence you would have broken the spell of silence you were under at an earlier time.

In today's world, people are busier when alone than with companions. They are busy with their phone, tablets, watches, even without these gadgets the mind is busier having a replay of an argument, a movie, a social media post or imagining a future event that may never occur. A time of silence also known as quiet time has been used more as a form of correction for children without really directing them on what to do during the quiet time.

A busy mind will never get anything new. It will only keep on replaying past problems and usual solutions. You need a silent time to get your creativity to a whole new level you or get a direction. There are so many benefits that can come from a time alone.

The gift of being alone is that you learn to belong to yourself first. It gives you a time to work on yourself, to fill your cup so you won't have to pour out of an empty cup. You must know who you are to be in the driver seat of your own life, not letting life drive you around without you knowing the destination. You will find true connection when you have first connected with yourself. If not, you risk the dangers of coming in contact with the consequences of belonging at all cost.

THE RISK OF BELONGING AT ALL COST

The more we want to belong to others the more we have the need for attention and approval, which often leads us to the disease called people pleaser. A disease is often associated with a medical condition but it simply means dis-eased, which means the sufferer is not at ease. Therefore, whatever makes you not at ease is a disease that could be cured. If you have ever suffered the people pleaser disease, rest assured you are not alone.

There are many people who would rather forego what they want because they want to be accepted by a diverse group of people, fit into a friendship circle or be loved by someone who truly may not even care about their existence.

According to Dr. Susan Newman, a New Jersey-based social psychologist people pleasers "want everyone around them to be happy and they will do whatever is asked of them. They put everyone else before themselves. For some, saying 'yes' is a habit; for others, it's almost an addiction that makes them feel like they need to be needed. This makes them feel important and like they're contributing to someone else's life."[8]

In terms of trauma survivors, most of us learned a maladaptive coping strategy of excessive submissiveness. This often places us in the people pleasing trap.

For a person who has felt like they are at a disadvantage in society either they have had their innocence forcefully taken from them, misjudged, lose their caregivers at an early age, they think they must please the people in their lives in order to work their way back into the heart of others or find a place to fit in that heart or quite simply just be accepted.

Stripped of originality

> An original is always worth more no matter how old and ugly it is.

The truth is in an attempt to do so, most of us unconsciously make people our obsession and twist our values for theirs. No one's identity is more important than yours. You were made an original. Why are you trying to become a counterfeit of another person? An original is always worth more no matter how old and ugly it is. At least it will sell as a vintage and vintages are always worth more than the latest brand anyway so why bother being a counterfeit?

Stop trying to please people who will never be pleased no matter what you do. Don't think if you compromise yourself and what you stand for it will make a person in your life happy. That is never going to work. Unless you realize that everyone is solely responsible for making themselves happy because their response is their responsibility, you will cross several boundaries to make someone happy, which will only leave you hurt. So, stop trying to please an unpleasable person.

Emptied first

In most cases, people try to please others at their expense. You can't be everything to everybody and you don't have to answer every question that you are asked. That is the main difficulty people pleasers face. They want everyone to be happy but don't realize that by doing what they do they put their own happiness on hold. In some cases, people avoid their self-care to attend to the needs of others.

It is evident in most relationships where we voluntarily take the position of being the caregiver to everyone in our lives. Out of the history of relational lack often arises the quest to fulfill that need in others. As such, most survivors do whatever it takes to make everyone they come across comfortable without looking into their own needs until they get to a point of exhaustion. This realization often comes when they are physically, emotionally, socially and spiritually drained of the partially full cup they have been pouring out from.

It is not selfish to do the one thing you desire most for yourself. The one thing that makes you emotionally relaxed. It could be reading, stretching, exercises, meditation, writing, just stopping for a deep breath, a glass of water or whatever it is. It is that one thing that once you get out of your mind, you feel energized once again. You go around your activities smiling in the face of hurt because you know before the world throws whatever it has on you, your mind is happy to receive it because you took care of it first.

Don't give up on yourself at the expense of whatever significant thing or person you have in your life. If you don't pay attention to yourself you will not be there for them either. I like to remind myself of the words of the flight attendants before a plane takes off the ground.

They always give a lecture on the importance of using the mask in an emergency landing situation. However, they always caution the passengers to wear their mask first before attending to the person next to them even if it is their dearly beloved one who may encounter some difficulties in fitting on their own mask. For sure you want to be alive to help others but if you want to continue pleasing others before yourself, you may not live to see the fruits of your labour.

Give yourself permission

Sometimes, you don't have to wait for someone to give you permission to do what you want to do or say what you want to say. Some people pleasers must wait for their spouses, parents, children, bosses, and even the government to give them a go-ahead on what they really need to do or point them at a direction even if that means giving up on their burning dream.

I know the government on that list may get you thinking, "How does that happen?" It is customary that sometimes the government comes up with a list of skills they are experiencing a shortage for and need people to fill those gaps. Some people may not have any passion for those jobs but because they are filled with pity and want to please the government, they go head on to get trained for those jobs and forfeit their dream jobs. I am so in support of patriotism but don't mistake pity for patriotism.

Just so you know, if you are an employee or planning to become one, most employers admit that they prefer their employees to be confident at handling situations and coming up with solutions to problems as opposed to waiting for someone to spell out the answers for them at every given opportunity. Being a people pleaser, though you mean well you might be mistaken for lack of confidence when all you intended to do was to get a go-ahead from your boss or supervisor.

Striving to get affirmation from people in authority over you may be an issue but an even greater problem is difficulties saying "no" when you need to say it for your own sake. Really, there is no harm in setting boundaries with all relationships in your life, be it friendship, emotional, career, parenting, or mentoring. There has to be a point where you clearly state that this is how far I can go so I will go no further than that.

It doesn't mean you are a bad person, it simply means you are making the right decisions for the benefit of the relationship. You wouldn't want to keep on giving your word and find yourself going to unhealthy lengths to honour your word or avoid betraying the trust of some significant people in your life because you couldn't deliver your promise maybe not at the expected time and place. It is better to say no than to put your reputation at stake.

Your opinion matters

Remember, nobody will ever say it like you do.

"They have said it all" or "That is exactly what I wanted to say." Does that sound familiar? Sometimes when we are among the few people left to contribute on a subject we tend to say words like that, simply because we don't want to keep others longer or perhaps we don't want to say something that will contradict the previous speaker's point so we just tend to agree on what others have said.

If that sounds like you, when you next find yourself in a position to speak up, please do. We are looking forward to hearing your interesting ideas. Remember, nobody will ever say it like you do. There is a certain twist to it that only you can bring to the table so please don't buckle it in there anymore. I and millions of people look forward to hearing from you. Don't underestimate your words.

While you're at it also remember that not everyone's idea is worth keeping. Don't just take every word that falls into your ears and implement them because "What will she say if she hears I dumped her ideas in the bin? That will break her heart." It is better to break her heart than to break your principles and excellence.

If you do not accept a person's principle, don't stick around to justify their actions. Cast out the fear of bailing out from someone whose actions are unacceptable to you. Don't stick around making excuses simply because you don't want someone to be angry at you. The actions could lead to a more disastrous outcome and you may not be around to tell the story. It may not be as easy as it sounds but be courageous enough to call a spade a spade and not a fork because that is what the other party will be more contented with.

I understand every relationship is different but instead of making excuses for the actions of others, seek professional help if necessary but don't just keep the conversation in your head, bring it out and be relieved to relive the relationship. Do whatever you need to do to cast off the burden.

Hyper-validation

A people pleaser could also constantly want people to gratify them. It is not just about outcomes going in their favour but they get unhealthily unhappy if they are not being noticed, given approval or attention. Everyone and everything gets your attention and impresses you.

You must have your self-worth and self-confidence. The most important person in your life that needs to be happy is YOU. Let your confidence come from your internal features, not external forces. Do the things you need to do to build up yourself, the things that will make you feel more confident. You may need to start listening to life-building messages to feed your mind, read books in the areas you want to grow, start a consistent exercise program, meditate or improve your communication skills. If you are confident in yourself, you will not need others to validate you to feel comfortable. Accept it if it comes, in the same way you accept it if it doesn't come.

Inner circle

Another thing worth considering is to change your social group; the people you hang around with if you realize they are people who make you feel awesome only if you do something for them or they do something for you. Some of us have found ourselves in the company of people whom we have to keep giving presents to, to fuel connection in the relationship. That is an example of a hazardous relationship that is consuming and not productive. Surround yourself with productive people.

You can break away from hazardous relationships by changing your response to them. If you are invited to a place you really don't want to go but feel you must impress that person, you can start by telling the person you will consider the invitation and get back with a response. That way, you give yourself time to process a more respectful answer without pleasing the person at your expense. In this digital age, you can take advantage of technology to text, email or message your response. It allows you to avoid the pressure of hastily agreeing with the person standing in front of you.

For someone who has never been a people pleaser, this might sound weird but consider a person who has been in the habit of saying "Yes" to everything. It is nerve-wracking to automatically answer 'no' to a request so why not start one step at a time. Every new habit takes time to build so try not to feel overwhelmed about your new response.

Bent principles

If you have been a person who has no principles to guide your actions, it could be time to come up with some. When you have principles stick to them, don't twist them around to accommodate another person's principles. It is okay to learn and adopt new principles but that is different from twisting your belief to please others. Understand what your beliefs are and follow them because that is where your honour resides. This will make it easier to say no to people and events that don't fit in with your principles, goals, vision, and schedule.

You won't have to apologize for sticking to your principles. Apologizing and complaining seems to be the norm of the day but it is time to kick it out of your life. Be fully responsible for the things that happen to you so you won't need to apologize to anyone if you fail or complain about why you were not able to wake up after the fall. When you seize maturity to be responsible for your successes and failures, you will realize you won't have to please people who truly don't care about what happens to you.

Rejection

It is okay to be rejected and it is okay to reject others. In fact, if you have a role model in your life, seek out time and have a conversation with that person. Ask just one question "Have you ever been rejected in your life?" I guarantee you the answer will be yes. Successful people have been rejected by employers, admirers, loved ones, and parents. I mean you are not alone. Everyone faces disapproval so don't continue letting yourself being manipulated and used for fear of rejection. Your integrity is more important than popularity.

It is okay to have an approval in your life just like there is a healthy amount of using some substances. However, don't let the approval dominate your life because that is where the problem lies. A lot of resources have been put in place to stop substance addiction. I am not against that but if we can put an end to approval addiction then a lot of other addictions will be eradicated as well.

It is time to eat what you want to eat, wear what you want to wear, go where you want to go, say what you want to say, meet who you want to meet, laugh when you want to laugh, cry when you want to cry, date who you want to date, the list goes on and on. That is how much lives have been stuck for the sake of others. You can do it if the new person you are creating fits into your principles and it's taking you closer to where you want your life to be in the future.

Stop caring about things that don't matter.

Don't get trapped in the lives of others and miss the route to who you want to be. Every person on Earth has a purpose but if you are trapped in the purpose of others, you miss the purpose for your own life. If there is someone you must fit into their purpose, it should be God's purpose for your life. He created you so His purpose for your life will be fulfilled. His purpose is your real purpose for your life. I say your real purpose because so many things could cloud our judgements of our purpose.

Be who God created you to be. If you don't know who you are ask Him, you are not just to check if you are doing right or wrong according to God's list because He truly doesn't care about that. He is more concerned with having a relationship with you. If you have not started on the path in that relationship with him, get up and talk to him now because He has been waiting for you to have a chat with Him.

If you are to take home one phrase from this chapter, it should be this: stop caring about things that don't matter. Don't beat yourself up if you feel alone or you feel accepted. Be good at accepting that you will not always fit in, so learn to manage when you feel like you belong and when you feel like you don't.

TRUE BELONGING

The question my teenage/young adult self is asking the adult me now is did I finally find belonging? My answer is this quote by Brené Brown, which has helped shape my perspective on belonging, "True belonging is a spiritual practice, and it is about the ability to find sacredness in both being a part of something but also the courage to stand alone." Yes! I did find where I belong.

I found the joy in the sacredness of being part of something, but I also found joy and courage in my ability to stand alone. The courage of being alone produced the strength of being part of something. One more thing, don't try to live your life trying to please everyone because it will only lead to frustration.

JOURNEY WITH KIKI

Moments of being alone, especially without her partner next to her were Kiki's most dreadful moments. Her idea of being in a relationship with someone meant they had to be together at all times except moments when one person is at work or has to be away from the other party for genuine reasons.

She had invested her full trust in her partner and had formed a high level of emotional and physical dependence on him to the extent that a break in proximity led to tension and fights in their home. The emotional dependence caused her to do whatever it took to please him. In her own description, the situation reached a point where she was extremely approval-seeking and criticism-horrified.

After an in depth discussion on this topic with her coach, she began to wonder if this could have been another reason why her husband started keeping late nights and eventually estranged their relationship. Of course, she is not responsible for his actions; her reflection came from the position of improving her quality of life. There could be a million reasons and no justifiable explanation for this action but such length of attachment by an adult could cause a wide range of reactions from anyone.

It was liberating for her to come to understand the healthy level of attachment in her relationship, the value of being alone. She maximized the moments she found herself just in the company of herself and the results of this quality time alone were astonishing.

REFLECTION

1. Have you ever felt that you have to succumb to the opinions of people despite your beliefs and values?
2. How did you break free from people-pleasing or how are you planning to break free from it?

3. What are some personal benefits you have experienced from being alone?
4. Did it take a while for you to understand that there is a blessing in being alone?
5. What advice can you give to someone who is unhealthily attached to a relationship in their life?

CHAPTER 8:
THE PURSUIT OF HAPPINESS

Happiness is when what you think, what you say, and what you do are in harmony." —Mahatma Ghandi

Many of us who have experienced trauma of some kind tend to have a misplaced definition of happiness except when we know it but do not see ourselves worthy of accommodating and accepting happiness. We do care about being happy but somewhere within us we think it is a mirage so why bother? In fact, happiness is not one of our priorities. We estimate happiness will come from that act of acceptance so we go the extra mile of wanting to belong and possess happiness in the process because at some point we realized that being happy and belonging walk hand in hand.

You may have figured out my problem; at a certain stage in my life, I wanted to be happy; truly happy not just appear to have it. I felt I had failed in several areas of my life in my early years, I sure knew what it meant to be sad because I had so much experience with that to the extent that I could give a full lecture on what it means to be sad but I had no clue what it meant to be happy because I had always appeared happy but never really felt happy.

IS SUCCESS HAPPINESS?

Success is not about exceeding the expectations of others. It is not about endorsement from others.

I had heard people say over and over that happy people are successful people so I started looking out for the things that could make me happy so I could be called a successful person. I didn't want to be called a failure my entire life; though no one called me this – at least not in my hearing. That didn't stop me from thinking I was failing drastically. I kept a smiling face as a cover for a sour heart.

In my early twenties, I thought it was time for me to focus on getting what I really desired because to me that is where my happiness dwelt. If I got it, certainly I will prove to others that I am successful.

Was I right? Certainly not! I was so focused on getting what I wanted, which could be a good thing but I wasn't doing it for myself. My intention of getting it was to prove a point to those who love me and those who had hurt me. What I didn't know is that success is not about exceeding the expectations of others. It is not about endorsement from others.

What I realized after achieving "my success" is that happiness through success comes only when you are satisfied with what you have done compared to what you should or could have done. It is about outclassing yourself. I didn't focus on trying to make my mistakes right, rather my focus was on proving myself to others and in a way competing with people who didn't know they were in a competition; unknown to me, I was running a one-man race.

Happiness in Competition
During our upbringing, in sporting activities, arts, academic and family settings we may have received a direct or indirect message to be better than someone else. This plunged us in that spirit of competition, with a constant quest of more ways to prove we are more skilled, have greater endurance or more intelligence than whoever we are in competition with.

However, when that anchor trauma occurred, it left us with the mindset that we do not measure up to anyone we may have been in competition with. As such, either we stop trying to bring out our best or we become more competitive. A famous music composer and educator Benjamin Zander once said, "It is dangerous to have our musicians so obsessed with competition, because they will find it difficult to take the necessary risks for themselves to be great performers." This is so true not only with regards to music but to all aspects of life because in the face of competition most people have the tendency to succumb to fear.

We have all gone through those negative experiences that caused us to fear to do the things we should be doing. The natural thing to do is to withdraw due to the fear of failure. However, another way to look at the situation is to find the opportunities in them to confront your fears. It could be a time to discover yourself; discover the things that truly make you happy and areas you need to invest your time and energy on.

When we focus on competing with another person, there is always that feeling of lack. Irrespective of how much we try to meet that need, something seems to be lacking and in our mind, when we fill that lack then we will be happy. How many of us know we shall never be able to meet that need as long as your focus is on another person. While you are trying to meet their standard they are raising the bar for their own benefit so you end up chasing their last prospect.

But if you turn it around to focus on yourself, then you will draw out more creativity from within you, which may have never known existed. Believe it or not, every person on Earth has different abilities. When you focus on competition, you become a counterfeit of someone else's ability while yours is being covered in dust.

The good news is that at any point you realize that you are an original version of your ability; you have the power to wake up, dust off your ability and let it produce the happiness you have been pursuing.

Happiness in Community

You may have thought for a while that happiness occurs in a community, I do agree with you on that, maybe not in the dimension you look at but yes true happiness could be found in a community.

There is a Chinese proverb: "If you want happiness for an hour, take a nap. If you want happiness for a day, go fishing. If you want happiness for a year, inherit a fortune. If you want happiness for a lifetime, help somebody." What I find remarkable in this proverb is that short-term happiness centres on what you do for yourself while long-term happiness comes from what you do for others.

In order to live a life full of happiness, we have to look beyond what we can do for ourselves into what we can do for others. This might not be new to you because at some point in life you may have come across the statement, "It is more profitable to give than to receive." However, what you probably didn't know is that in the well of those words lies a significant key to happiness.

I do understand that giving services, time or possessions is not something that comes naturally for anyone, particularly not from a trauma survivor. That makes sense because something has been forcefully taken from you. As such why would someone who parted with something without their consent want to be in a position of vulnerability where they could likely be taken advantage of?

That notwithstanding, if you ever come to harmony with yourself where you can give back to humanity, you will realize that whenever you give you are not doing it for the benefit of the receiver as you may have thought all along; it is for your benefit. It might sound weird but it is the truth.

The act of offering any form of service to humanity is an opportunity to plant your interest and skills while filling the needs of others. I guess we do not need to be an award-winning farmer to know that any seed sowed at the right time will produce fruit.

I bet everyone is happy when they harvest the good fruits of their labour. It may not come in the form you expect but the reward will be greater than your expectation. When you put a smile on the face of someone, you put a stamp of joy in your heart. I love what Brendon

Burchard said, "You don't have happiness, you have to generate happiness. You don't have joy, you generate joy." You reap more than what you sow!

Happiness in Content

There is a high probability that whatever the traumatic experience is, it left you dissatisfied with certain aspects of your life. It could be a present or past living condition, family situation, environmental factors, physical appearance and/or emotional well-being.

If you look around the world today, it is evident that every part of the earth has different climatic seasons though some parts have two seasons while others have four. This only goes to show that though we may not all have the same experiences we all encounter a change in seasons.

The happiness we seek will be attained if we embrace the current season of life without waiting to be happy when we are in the next season. What I find most often is that we tend to not fully embrace the moment because we are focused on mourning the past or worried about the future. I understand there are moments when some trauma survivors experience flashbacks of abuse, violence and assault; that is entirely different from when we voluntarily replay in our minds the events of the past yet we hope to live in a state of happiness.

There are some things in life we do not have control over. For example, you can't change the season you are in from winter to spring or from rainy to dry season but you can change how you handle the unfavourable climate by making a choice to have the resources you need to minimize stress in the season.

If you are not excited about the course of your life up to this point, you can get the resource of being genuinely content in your present circumstances. This is not because your life is perfect. Hello! I wonder if anyone has that perfect life. It simply means you make a choice to be happy irrespective of what may be going on, in and around you.

The people you see whom you think are perfect may simply just be satisfied in the current season of their lives. You can too! You can choose to have that satisfaction while you look forward to getting what you desire.

> **Being in a state of contentment means you reconcile with your past, you commit to your present and redesign your future.**

The urge to make everything perfect robs the happiness that can be found in contentment. You may have had a chaotic past so right now you are doing everything you can to make the present and future perfect – as a result, you live in a constant state of burnout.

It is important to have goals, it is great to pursue them but it is best to find your balance. In other words, be content in every season of your life but don't get attached to a specific season because it will also change. Contentment is not a gift endowed on a few; it is a skill that everyone who desires it can develop.

Being in a state of contentment means you reconcile with your past, you commit to your present and redesign your future. You can have the present and future you desire and deserve. It starts within you and flows outward. Make a choice today to be content despite the circumstances you are in. That is the solution to getting out of it. When you are happy, you attract more events, which will bring more happiness into your life.

Happiness in Character?

One thing I learned is that happiness is a choice. It is not dependant on my circumstances; it is dependent on my choices. I am responsible for my happiness, not my husband, not my children, not my job, not the economy, not my health, but me.

So then if I am responsible for my own happiness what do I have to focus on? The answer I got was a shock to me: "Focus on developing yourself and build your integrity." Don't wait for someone to make you happy and don't try to change someone. Make a choice to be happy and change yourself then everything will come into place.

In most situations, the problem doesn't lie in other people but in our perspective. I found out that character and choices are the most important tools needed to succeed. This is why I agree with Jim Rohn when he said, "Success is something you attract by the person you become." The choices you make account for the person you are becoming.

If you build your character and stick to it you will avoid most of the problems that are affecting your life negatively. Things like peer pressure will have no effect on you. A person of character is a person who lives by principles. This person is built on a solid foundation and therefore will not sway in every direction the wind pushes.

Back to the example of peer pressure. If a friend comes to you and requests to share a substance with you that you don't consume and you had built your life on the principle never to operate in a substance-induced state, that problem will be easy to solve. You simply tell your friend using such substances is against my principles so I won't take it.

You might be ridiculed, mocked and called names but it is expected. Every person of character has had that experience but they remain at peace because their joy comes from sticking to who they have chosen to be. In the long run, when your character is known among your peers the pressure will be taken off you because your peers know your limits so they know what you get involved in and what you stay away from. It all starts with a choice.

A person of character is unwavering. It is not a person who makes a choice today then does something different tomorrow. This means how you are known in private should be the same person you are in public. A dual lifestyle is the cause of many frustrations. This doesn't mean you should wash all your linens in public, it simply means if you have chosen to be happy, do whatever it takes to maintain your happiness in private as you do in public. Don't come out to the world as a happy, jovial person but when you get home you return to the sad, grumpy person. All that does is set in confusion, which leads to chaos in your life. If you truly have reasons to be unhappy, look for solutions to the problems so you can take off that cap for good rather than living in pretense.

It is like the life of most celebrities or politicians. People love their music, acting or campaigns but often get disappointed at some point in their career because their character is different from charisma. With time, fans and followers discover that the person is not what they expected them to stand for. Without being judgemental, today we find many high profile personalities who seem to have it all then watch everything go down the drain due to the consequences of living a double life. That should not be the case, let your integrity be the bedrock for your actions.

A person of character is whole. I am not the best at Math, but just in case you are like me and wondering about the meaning of integrity, in my quest for the meaning I learned that it comes from the word integer which means complete in itself – wholeness. Who would have thought math would interfere in how I live my life but here it is a very powerful undeniable force.

"Wholeness does not mean perfection: it means embracing brokenness as an integral part of life."—Parker J. Palmer.

Let's face it, our life will never be problem free but when we embrace the broken pieces; allowing ourselves to be vulnerable because we are true to the real selves, that to me is integrity. It doesn't mean you are perfect, it means you are mindfully being you.

You must be the same wherever you are, with everyone you meet. A group of people should not know you as one person while another group knows you as another person. Have you ever heard your friends/ the media/social media posts talking about someone you know and deep within your heart you're wondering if they're referring to the same person because the description they're giving doesn't fit with the person you know?

If you have, I'm sure that made you feel betrayed irrespective of whether the person is a close or a distant relation. You were either betrayed because the person has been misrepresented or betrayed because you saw a real side of the person you never knew existed. Choosing integrity comes with the benefit of peace because it relieves the burden of trying to cover up for deeds caused by the other side of you.

A person of character is predictable. The people around you know what you can say or do and therefore they can trust you to work with. You might say I don't want to be predictable because that makes me vulnerable. Well I have news for you, unless you are predictable you will never have true friends or followers because no one wants to invest their heart in a wavering soul. Trust is only built on a foundation of integrity.

> Your self-confidence will be boosted when you start practicing being a person of integrity.

It also comes with a benefit of confidence. Your self-confidence will be boosted when you start practicing being a person of integrity. You will not have to panic when you meet someone you are trying to hide a portion of your life from. When your phone rings, you won't have to contemplate what to tell the caller because you're trying to catch up with the last information you gave. It will keep you in a relaxed state while you live out loud.

If you are wondering if you have integrity or have come to a place like I did where I made a choice to be a person of integrity, you may want to look at these three steps, which worked for me as well as others I know who are people of character.

Firstly, you have to trust in something/someone bigger than you.
Let's be honest, our nature is very unstable. We want to do one thing but end up doing another without being able to explain what transpired between our intentions and our actions. Therefore, we cannot truly be a person of integrity on our own. We need a more solid foundation to build on.

You need a force that is greater than what you can control. I made a choice at some point in my life to trust in God. I had known Him my whole life but I never had a relationship with Him. I knew Him as a deity, which is one way to know Him, but I discovered that for me to really know Him I had to discover another side of Him; the person part of Him. He offers an invitation for us to trust in Him. This invitation comes up several times in His conversation through the Bible that you can't miss. So, I decided to put my trust in Him while adopting His ways as the base of my character.

While I trust in God, I also like to ask myself if the choices I make prepare me for a life in eternity. I set my mind on eternity not because I need a perfect performance to receive a crown of life but because I need to set my heart in a position where I am at peace with myself, so I do not take for granted the grace that has been offered to me.

Secondly, look for a role model.
Surround yourself with the right people. It could just be someone whose lifestyle inspires you and demonstrates who you want to be; someone whose principles you can emulate. You may not be exactly like that person in one day, one year, ten years or forever but as you continue learning from that person you gradually change from the old habits you want to discard and adopt the new habits you want to exemplify. A role model guides you, corrects you, and affirms you. You may even have a model whom you have never met in person but by you just reading about them, listening to them speak you are changed into who you desire to be.

> *A good role model will not always pamper your flaws but will also chisel your character.*

When you do find that person, don't pretend to have your act all together. Maintain your true identity in the process of learning to improve yourself. When you pretend to be your mentor your focus will be in yourself, on how well you are keeping up to being who are not as oppose to learning to become who you want to grow into.

Finally, be ready to fail forward.
There will be moments of mistakes. I did and I still do fail as well as a host of others I know but what matters is for your heart to focus on the

right direction; to have a repentant heart that will rise from the fall with a determination to make it right.

In John Maxwell's words, "The more you do, the more you fail. The more you fail, the more you learn. The more you learn, the better you get." No one ever got it right the first time and no one is failure proof. Integrity just like happiness is not optional, it is a must have, a must keep, a must practice. It is a life-changing key to unlocking the cage so you can thrive. A key that is found in your hands and only you can use it to unlock your own doors.

ABOVE ALL: BOUNDARIES!

When I think of boundaries, the story of Dr. Jill Bolte Taylor as told by Oprah Winfrey in *The Wisdoms of Sundays* (page 327–329) comes to mind. During recovery from a hemorrhagic stroke, which affected the functioning of her left hemisphere and made her intensely aware of the energy in her surroundings, Dr. Jill said, "There were only two types of people in the world: those who bring energy and those who drain." She went on to make a sign which reads, "Please take responsibility for the energy you bring into this space."

The principle of boundaries is one that should never be neglected in any relationship by a person who desires a life of happiness. This may not be something you are accustomed to especially if you had your mental, physical, social or spiritual possessions infringed on by someone you once trusted. However, in any kind of relationship you find yourself in, it is imperative to set a limit for a healthy relationship with yourself and others. You have to be keenly aware of the people in your life and the energy they deposit into you.

The energy people carry doesn't always stay with them. When you come into contact with any person, if you are not mindful of your feelings you may end up picking up the energy of the other person. Make sure you surround yourself with the best so you don't become a dumping ground for garbage.

TWO-STEP PROCESS

- The first step in setting boundaries is having self-awareness. Knowledge of yourself will help you realize the things that awaken negative emotions in you. This will guide you on your limits and what not to allow in your space.
- Secondly, recognize that you matter. Failure to register this recognition in your mind will lead you to think that you are being selfish by setting boundaries in your life. Inasmuch as happiness can be generated when we offer service to humanity, sadness can also be generated when it comes from a position of guilt and resentment. You have a right to say "yes" or "no" when necessary, so exercise it.

Before you spontaneously agree to commitments, criticisms or advice, think about yourself. Take into consideration the feeling you will get if you follow through with the commitment, advice or criticism.

JOURNEY WITH KIKI

Happiness had always been a stranger in Kiki's life. She so much desired it but didn't know how to generate it. As a child, she so much depended on her parents to make her happy. This seems to be the norm because most children look up to their caregivers and often have their emotions guided by them. However, what happens when the people your happiness is dependent upon inflict so much physical and emotional pain on you?

Despite the physical pain her father inflicted on her via sexual abuse and the emotional pain she constantly experienced each time her mother blamed her for alluring her father's actions then cautioning her to keep the "family secret", she still thought they kind of made her happy when they showered her with gifts; things her peers only dreamed about.

However, when the sources of her happiness vanished from the earth, she knew she had lost every reason to be happy so she became all too familiar with sadness.

She lit the candle of happiness once more in her life after she tied the knot with her man. Although she had not felt genuinely happy for a long time, somehow she just thought this man was going to make her happy. So she picked up this candle and for years she searched for the happiness she expected. When she didn't get it from this source, she later turned to her children after their birth.

Just like in her marriage, she experienced a glimpse of her pursuit in the first few months of the relationship but the candlelight grew dimmer with each passing day until it finally went off, leaving her in a deeper realm of sadness; what she described as depression.

Thanks to her concerned mommy friend who introduced her to therapeutic relationships, she came to realize that true happiness comes from within. One of its sources is unlocking your potential and engaging your skills in what you are passionate about.

It had always been her desire to offer some sort of help to girls who have experienced female genital mutilation. Her push factor was the pain during and after the process, the health issues she had experienced later in life which she associated with it, not leaving out the fact that her father had linked his act on her "maturity" after her circumcision.

She knew she had to be a voice to many who, like her, had been silenced by the perpetrators of the deed. She knew many who needed a friend, a mentor, a coach, a counselor or a therapist; a person she never knew could help her until she found herself in the life-changing relationship.

She just wanted to hold a peer's hand, smile at them and say, "I understand your experience! I am here for you! You are not alone!"

This marked the beginning of her volunteer activities with an organization dedicated to advocating the prevention of gender-based violence such as breast and belly ironing, female genital mutilation, rape, and incest. They also train women on sexual and reproductive health as well as coach and counsel survivors of abuse. With her involvement in this work, she began to experience what true happiness feels like.

She made a choice to go a step further by identifying her principles. When she had a clear picture of them, she came up with a plan and set the ball rolling on creating appropriate barriers in her life, in order to guard her newfound positive energy.

REFLECTION

1. How do you define happiness?
2. In your opinion, what creates happiness?
3. Which periods in your life do you identify as the times you felt happiest? Can you pinpoint the nature of activities or relationships present in your life at that time?
4. What areas in your life do you currently feel happy about? What lessons can you identify in those areas which you can apply to have an overall genuine happiness?
5. What areas in your life are you unhappy about? What changes can you make to transcend from unhappiness to happiness in that area?

Irrespective of the state you are in know that you can produce something out of nothing. You have the power to make your life what you want it to be!

CHAPTER 9:
TURNING POINT

"I am here for a purpose and that purpose is to grow into a mountain, not to shrink to a grain of sand. Henceforth will I apply ALL my efforts to become the highest mountain of all and I will strain my potential until it cries for mercy."
—Og Mandino

Have you been waiting for so long, **really** hoping for things to just fall into place in your life? Waiting for the dream job to be offered to you, waiting for that relationship to just work out the way you want it to be, or waiting for that physical, emotional pain to vanish with time; after all, it is said: "Time heals all wounds." Are you waiting for time to manifest its supernatural powers in your favour?

You know, there is something about the mindset that everything that has to come into your life will just fall into place. Do you ever wonder how you came about with that idea? Well I did, because it was a predominant force in my mind. If you are like me, at one point in your life, through words and/or actions you were made to believe that you have no control over the circumstances of your life. That is the answer to why you believe everything will come into place.

I was okay with that mindset until I heard a statement that "There are two great days in a person's life; the day you were born and the day you discover why you were born." That means the reason you were born doesn't come automatically on the day of your birth. So if it doesn't come automatically why should I think everything I desire will come with time?

Before this time, I had never really considered why I was born beside of course at one point I had thought I was born to be a victim of negative circumstances of some sort. When I found out that was a lie, I discarded that knowledge of myself but still couldn't figure out the purpose for my existence.

Following the season of my bliss; of the new beauty around me when I began picking out the lies, dropping and replacing them with the truth came a time when I felt dissatisfied, not because I wasn't happy but there was a lingering desire that I was made for more so I have to discover more about myself.

Self-love is not selfishness, it is a necessity

There was a lack of conviction that I had discovered why I was born. I felt selfish because I was getting what I always wanted so why would I think there was more to me than what I was getting? Note that self-love is not selfishness, it is a necessity. The truth is I had never had a relationship with myself to the extent of knowing what I truly wanted.

Up until this point, I had been floating by a force without really knowing what direction my life was heading so I decided to embark on the journey to discover myself. One would have thought that getting traditional education would lead to this discovery but I may have missed that lesson at some point in school.

It is very important to get formal education but very dangerous if you acquire it to a certain level without knowing who you are because you might be purchasing knowledge you do not need. Any knowledge not put into use is not worth getting. An accurate knowledge of your purpose is the most important information you need to get.

PULL IT OUT

Purpose is a steering wheel of life, it will lead you on what courses to study, what books to read, what kind of music to listen to. So, I knew

I had to get that knowledge of myself since I had never learned it in school. I thought I was educated but when my education did not give me what I wanted I decided to dive deeper to find out the meaning of education. It turns out the word education like many English words come from the Latin word *educere*, which means to draw out.

If education means to draw out that means there is something stuck within somewhere. So my question is what lies within? Many of the encounters we experienced have cluttered what we have within us. In order to find what lies within, you will have to do some decluttering.

> In order to find what lies within, you will have to do some decluttering.

We all have our dreams or at least we did at some point, we envisioned our lives turning out in a certain way but oftentimes who we think we are is actually not who we really are. I have had dreams of totally unrelated careers. Not just dreaming about them but taking steps to see how it could become a reality before asking myself, "Really! Is that what you want to do? Is that who you are?"

Your purpose could be covered in circumstances if you knew what it is at a point in your life. On the other hand, if like me, who was still to discover what it is, the reason could be that we have abandoned our true nature. Some people have abandoned their purpose to become a photocopy of another person thereby losing their self and others have just believed the lies from people and external influence.

It is pretty common to have such outcomes since most of us are so focused on some celebrities and trying to be like them to the extent that we are not true to own selves. This can happen if you are focused so much on yourself that you fail to realize that life is not just about you getting what you want but making an impact in the lives of others and the world at large.

What I mean by focusing on you is that sometimes we just want to be like another person for our personal interest. Your real purpose is bigger than me, myself and I. Your purpose is about making a difference! One thing I discovered about human nature is that when it dawns on you that you are making an impact in one life you will have a thirst to impact even more people through the minute and grand decisions you make.

When the attention is only on you, it makes you indifferent and ineffective in your relationship with others. What often happens is you will embrace what they have for you, what they can do for you but fail to see what is in you so you might end up chasing what others have.

Stop waiting for someone to bring something to you that is already inside of you. You could be looking up to a designer to find out the latest design they will release so you can be a billboard for them whereas somewhere within you lies a person who was made to come up with something the world may never see if you don't stop focusing on others so you can see the treasure in you.

I once heard Dr. Myles Munroe say, "The wealthiest places in the world are not the gold mines, oil fields, diamond mines or banks. The wealthiest place is the cemetery. There lies companies that were never started, masterpieces that were never painted … There is a treasure within you that must come out. Don't go to the grave with your treasure still within you." He also went on to say, "The greatest tragedy in life is not death, but a life without a purpose." Those words haunted me so much and left me seeking the answer to one question.

WHAT IS PURPOSE?

When children get to the age of communicating in sentences, usually around the ages of 3–5 years old, most caregivers can't help feeling overwhelmed around them due to the continuous stream of why questions that flow out of their mouths. Questions like, why is the sky blue? Why do we have rocks on the ground? Why are there stars in the sky? Why do I have to sleep at night? Why … why … why?

The problem is they often ask the questions to people whom they assume have all the answers that exist but ironically, these adults don't even have the answer to the most important why, which is the why of their own lives though unlike the children they are not bold enough to ask the question or they have asked the wrong source.

Your purpose is something you were created to do. What that says is if you do something outside of what you are created to do you will never have satisfaction doing it. If you have had the good fortune to know so many people in this world, you may have come across people who have more degrees than a thermometer, have amassed so much wealth, and are the envy of others who are trying to attain a certain level of their "success" yet those people are extremely unsatisfied in their lives.

The reason is often that they have been functioning outside of their purpose. They could be succeeding at what they do but that doesn't mean they are living their purpose.

Everything in life has a purpose so everything you do should have a purpose. Before you engage in any activity or a relationship, in order to have fulfillment in it, it is imperative for you to know the purpose of it before commencement. The reason I can tell you this is because many of the failures I have experienced in my life is because I got into associations that had no defined purpose, but I felt I had to please someone or more than one person.

Besides human beings, every created thing knows its nature and sticks to it. I believe the reason most human beings don't operate within their purpose is that they have the ability to think and make a choice so they choose to debate the truth even without a conviction that they have reasons to debate.

The flowers know they must produce nectar, the bees know they have to collect nectars to make honey. You will never see a bee trying to produce nectar nor a flower producing honey but not so with humans. We often drift from our purpose, use things out of the prescribed usage, do not follow the due order and as such don't do things the right way, leading to a new order of abuse.

THE ORIGIN OF ABUSE

When things are not used according to the plan of the creator we call it abuse. The word abuse is said to originate from a Latin word *abuti* – ab(away) uti(to use) – which means something has been taken away from its original purpose to be used in a different manner. In other words, it is abnormally used.

While in college, I had a course called abnormal psychology. Personally, I found this title very disturbing because it gave me an initial idea that what I was going to study would be something different from normal psychology. In my growing mind, I couldn't figure what is normal and abnormal psychology. Studying the course didn't clarify my worries about the course title though I learned some great stuff.

Unlike my course, there are several things that are abnormally used. Just because something you do works doesn't mean you are fulfilling the purpose of it. Just because you are in a position to have sex with a vulnerable person doesn't mean you are fulfilling the purpose of sex. That is why it is said you are abusing the person.

I say this respectfully; all sorts of addictions are driving well-meaning people to do things out of their reasoning capacity. If everything is used within its required dosage to fulfil its purpose, there will be so much relief from most of the social problems society encounters. That is how important purpose is to us.

PURPOSE IN PERSPECTIVE

You can't guess the purpose of a thing, the only secure way to find out is to ask its manufacturer. There are over a billion users on Facebook today but if you really want to know why it was created you have to ask the creator. That is the only source that will reveal what they had in mind before it saw the light of day. So many Facebook accounts have been blocked; other users have been sued because of their activities on Facebook simply because they failed to use it according to its purpose. They abnormally used it from the original intention of the creator so their actions brought in consequences.

The same applies to the Internet. Some say it is the best thing that happened to this generation because it has brought the world together more than any other time in history yet the mother who lost a child to suicide from online bullying might not share the same idea of "the Internet being the best thing for this generation." Does that mean the

Internet is bad? Absolutely not! Some people just choose to use it outside the purpose of the manufacturer.

You can guess ten or more reasons why I am writing this book but if you want to know the purpose of the book, you will have to get into my mind; you will have to ask me. Any information not coming from me will be assumptions. Sometimes you can guess and get the winning ticket but how many people win the lotto in a year? Your life is greater than a lottery system, don't gamble with it.

Why were you born in this time and age? Why weren't you born in the first century or in the twenty-fifth century? Why now? There is a purpose for you being on Earth this day and time. There is something that only you can accomplish. There is something that flows naturally from you. Bring into the world what has been deposited in you.

Every part of your life has a purpose. There is a purpose for you to be a child, there is a purpose for you to a sibling, there is a purpose for you to be a spouse, there is a purpose for you as a parent, and there is a purpose for you to be an employer, an employee, a business owner, a minister. An attempt to take your purpose for being a child and impose it on your purpose for being a spouse might cause your system of marriage to crash. Find out the purpose for every component of your life.

If you decide to start a business, what is your purpose for starting that business? Is it for you to compete with others in that business? Is it for you to show your former employer that you can be a better boss? You must establish a purpose for starting that business before you fling its doors open to the public; if not you are heading the wrong direction from day one.

> *To me, purpose is when your instincts, your honesty, your wholeness in yourself tells you that what you are doing is right. You find fulfillment, accomplishment and an overall worthiness to the extent that no matter what anyone says to you, you know without an iota of doubt that you are doing what you were made to do.*

BRINGING IT HOME

The greatest thing about what you have in life is why you have it. The root cause of social problems, as well as some health and economic problems, is that most people have pursued what they want without knowing why they want it. I can attest to that because that is part of my story.

The two days that marked our marriage celebration are ones beyond words. A part of me was super excited while another part of me was like, really? In case you are wondering if I really meant to say two days, doubt no more, the answer is yes. Just so you know if you are not already aware, most African marriages are commemorated in two or three celebrations depending on if you have a traditional, civil and church wedding and how you schedule the occasions. Notwithstanding, most of the activities are spread out on two or more days. So, my two days celebration was one of the shortest celebrations.

Glowing in the glamour of the day, enjoying the status of being the centre of attraction, smiling to several photographers whom I still wonder the outcome of the pictures taken, feeling fabulous in the most beautiful dress I believe I have ever worn, but not without doubt, on the highest heels I have ever had on and confident in well decorated hair accompanied by perfectly done make-up, yet I wasn't sure of what I was getting into.

The pressure of finding the answer to that question was not so much at the civil marriage as it was during the traditional marriage. One year earlier, I had attended a traditional marriage ceremony where the parents of the bride told the bride they were not going to use the money and items paid as bride price in case the marriage doesn't work out and they would have to pay back to the groom the items and money they had received as the bride price.

In that situation, the parents were not convinced their daughter had passed their test to have a successful marriage so though they were giving her to a man in marriage, they had their fingers crossed that she might come back to them. That may have given me some assurance if that was my scenario because then I would have known I am not the only person not sure of what I was going into but there are others who shared my thoughts and would receive me back with open arms saying, "I am not surprised."

A few friends and relatives had aired their sentiments about me being too young to get married though I am not sure if there is a right age. Some will say a person is too young to get married and others will say a person is getting too old to get married so I smiled through their sentiments.

Nevertheless, as I stood there looking at my prince charming whom I couldn't wait to be called his wife, I couldn't help asking myself, "Why am I getting married" and "What does marriage mean to me by the way?" Strange enough before now, I thought I knew all the answers from the movies, the books but I had never personalized this question so why now? Why at a time when I believed there is no going back?

My problem was not the person I was getting married to. My problem was the institution of marriage. My beloved biological father passed away when I was eight years old. As a child, I never had an example of what marriage is about. Later as a preteen, I went to live with my grandmother who was blessed to still have my grandfather with her.

The thing is my grandmother was in a polygamous marriage so the drama in the home is another story altogether. If there was one thing I learned from that relationship it was never to get into a polygamous marriage. However, one of the greatest miracles I have witnessed is that today we are all a big happy family.

Years into my marriage, I still didn't know the purpose of marriage. I had my expectations and a long list of things I wanted my marriage to look like but my disappointment led to frustration. To make matters worse, my dilemma became double fold with the birth of my children. Not only could I not answer the question of why I was married, but I also did not know why I am a mother either. I still had my list of expectations, which had now doubled because I added the expectations for my children.

The whole situation got more confusing because nothing was going my way. I had a daughter before who was practically raised by everyone besides me. So here I am, almost a "new mom" who is new in another country. Besides my husband, I had no family members to guide me in raising the kids so I either find out my purpose as a mother and wife or I keep gambling with those important relationships in my life.

This was the beginning of another quest for knowledge. The day I got the revelation of my purpose as a mother and a wife was truly one of the most important days of my life. That brought me closer to understanding the general purpose of my life.

The reason I shared this slice of my life with you is to let you know that wherever you are at, at the moment, it is not too late or too early to go after your purpose. Winston Churchill said, "It's not enough to have lived. We should be determined to live for something." What are you determined to live for?

In my case, I found my purpose by consulting my creator through talking to Him and reading the manual for my life and listening to Him talk back to me through any channel He chooses. A practice of stillness and meditation helped me to find the answers, which had always been within me.

The only way to find out the purpose for your life is to ask your creator. I cannot tell your purpose, I didn't manufacture you; perhaps someone else on Earth can do that but, the only source I know is your source. I can guide you on how to discover it for yourself, help you to develop it but you are the only person to discover and affirm the exact purpose of your existence. There are some clues to look out for while developing your purpose. However, what I find with most people is that purpose is something which flows out of you naturally.

PASSION VS PURPOSE

Passion and purpose are interconnected but don't confuse your passion for your purpose. In my experience, I have had several things I am passionate about at a moment but after a while of pursuing them, I lost my passion for those things. However, with purpose, you have an aura of fulfillment each time you do something within your purpose. That sensation just keeps building higher the more you develop your skills in the area of your purpose.

That notwithstanding, it is important to look out for the things that absorb your attention. Listen to your inner self and follow your instinct. Sometimes the things you really want to do may be different from what you have studied in school your entire life. Develop the areas of your passion for your treasure could be where your heart lies.

You could be passionate about several things so don't get anxious if there are several things running through your mind because you may have heard that there is just one thing you are passionate about. I have met people who have several passions, which sometimes all boils down to one purpose.

I have often heard that your passion is something you can do for free at any hour of the day. That is right to an extent; I have also discovered that you can discover your passion through what you are doing at the moment. There is no defined method to find your passion because what works for one person might not work for the next. So, feel free to explore your options but if you find your purpose during your passion, don't let it go.

Some have found their passion in giving their full force and energy to their current project. Does that mean passion is something that can be developed? Absolutely! You need to fan the flames of your passion in order to take it to the level where you can give it your all and fall in the category of those who say passion is something you can do for free at any time of the day if that is what you want passion to mean to you.

Most people I know have fuelled passion by solving their problems and those of others. In other words, if you are the kind of person who sits and waits for things to come to you, this might not be for you. I believe you fuel your passion by going out on adventures be it in your career, relationships, or personal life.

Look for new ways to do the things you love to do and while you're at it, have fun helping people along the way. Bring in your energy to fuel the needs of someone who is weak in that area. Your passion is more useful when you use your strengths to bring balance to a place of weakness along the path of your talents.

GIFTS VS ABILITIES

A gift has been given to you. There is no person walking the earth who has never been given a gift even if you have never received one physically.

At Christmas, birthdays, special occasions, you may have received a gift from a well-meaning person who got something for you thinking it might just be what you need. What happens often is that when we open the packaging, what we see is not always what we had expected to receive, except in recent times where I see people releasing a list of their needs prior to their special days.

Unlike physical gifts, God has given every one of us spiritual gifts. Some have received theirs, opened them and are utilizing them. Others have received their gifts but are still to open the package; some do not even know there is a gift with their name on it.

Amongst the many things you are great at doing; your gift is the thing you do extremely well with the least amount of effort. An artist could paint a picture without formal training and everyone who sees the image can't hold back their appreciation for the beautiful work of art. You may have listened to some untrained singer sing, and the music penetrates deep into your soul leaving you wondering if you just heard an angel's voice.

Another person may not have the ability to get that initial wow factor, but because they desire that ability, they go the extra mile in an effort to develop a talent they might have for singing. Some have called spiritual gifts natural talent because unlike someone who develops their abilities a gift flows naturally though it gets better with practice.

Many times, we are pushed into areas that are not in the area of our gifts. Yes! We have remarkable results doing it but the fact that a decorative bowl can be used for soup doesn't mean it is doing what only it can do. There is a certain beauty that bowl can bring into the world, which will never be achieved otherwise if we keep putting soup in it.

Some have abandoned their gifts because they listen to opinions that directed them to follow their abilities to areas which they believe will produce more money, more influence or more popularity. Pursue your gift!

For some people, they may have to dig deeper into their spirit to find their gift. It is often not hard to find it. The problem often lies in the fact that they haven't taken time to think about it but they may be using their gift at a certain level without realizing it.

> *Don't let the lies you have been told about yourself blur your gift. Use it; it will take you to places you never thought possible.*

EMBRACING IT

Once you have found your purpose, your gift, what you are passionate about; embrace it - don't let it go. As simple as it may sound it is not often easy for some to embrace it. It may require leaving your comfort zone, walking away from what you have done your entire life yet it is the one thing you can do like no one else, without struggling to make it a masterpiece. In the process of embracing it, you have to love yourself and value other people.

It is easy to say, "I love you" to someone in our lives though sometimes we really don't mean what we say, don't know why we say it but decide to flow with the formality. Sometimes after saying it repeatedly, we get to start loving the people or come to an understanding of the real meaning of the phrase.

Let's be honest, it sounds egocentric for me to say I love myself yet that is the realization you must come into to fully embrace your purpose. A few people may question, "What does she think she is?" "Who is she anyway?" "Do you hear the way she talks about herself?" "How dare she say she loves herself?"

Let those words come in one ear and leave through the other, maybe that is the purpose for having two ears, I am not sure. What I am certain is that when you love yourself, you will not betray yourself. Many have betrayed who they are, betrayed their purpose to fit into what society or their caregivers want them to be.

Some children have taken different paths from their purpose because they feel indebted to their parents for raising them, so they think they have to pay back that debt by becoming who their parents want them to be.

> **Be true to yourself and walk away. You can fulfil your purpose in another environment that will help your seed flourish.**

Others are functioning in the area of their purpose in an environment that causes them to undervalue themselves. In the process they may not be getting the fulfillment they know they deserve; others may be experiencing emotional, physical, or psychological abuse. Yet they are betraying themselves by sticking to that environment. Be true to yourself and walk away. You can fulfil your purpose in another environment that will help your seed flourish.

You can easily know when you are betraying yourself because it will cost you emotional energy; it will drain you of all the motivation you need to move forward. When you are tired, your physical energy has depreciated. There are instances when you are exhausted physically but you can keep going, keep pushing on because you tap into your inner energy to refuel your physical body. But when you are drained internally, the flow does not go from the outside in; it has to be from the inside out. You don't need to be a person of faith or a religious person to have an internal part. We all have it. What matters is what you do to make it come alive.

When you betray yourself, you lose yourself and risk losing your life. You may still be living – spirit, soul and body – but you find that you are just existing and not living. I once heard someone say, "Some people died at twenty but they were buried at sixty-five." That is because they betrayed themselves at twenty and kept on living till they were declared dead by a medical practitioner at sixty-five. If others betray you, you can bounce back but if you betray yourself, it only takes the grace of God to recover yourself. Thank God that grace is sufficient for us all.

IT'S BEYOND YOU

I am still to meet someone who will tell me that their purpose is just for them, someone to tell me that they do not need to connect with other people in the process of accomplishing it.

Imagine what would happen if Steve Jobs had stayed in his house, designed the iPhone, kept it on his shelf and stared at it all day without sharing the creation with a single soul. As I write this, I wonder how he could have created the phone if he didn't go out to get the materials created by another person of purpose, which he needed to create the idea he had in mind.

He had a purpose, he had a passion, and he had a gift but it would have been buried with him if he didn't market it to valuable customers. The world would never have seen a product exactly like the products he created. Another person may have designed something, but it would never have been the same.

There is an African proverb which says, "A single tree cannot make a forest." Another proverb says, "One hand cannot tie a bundle." That is an emphasis on teamwork. There is a certain level of your purpose you may be able to accomplish by yourself. You may just need a quiet time to develop that idea running through your mind, but you need others if you have to take it to the next level.

This is why you need to have a true value for people irrespective of what you have experienced. Many retail businesses and restaurants have customer appreciation day. Is it because they have excess products and don't know what to do with them, so they decide to give them away for free or at lower prices? No! Every true leader knows that people will work with you in accomplishing your purpose if you show them you truly value the relationship you have with them.

Many countries in the world at one point have cried out for help to oust a dictator. Others took the matters into their hands to devise methods to solve the problem. Amongst the many reasons for these actions, if the people had been treated by their leaders as valuable, they may have worked with them to accomplish the intended purpose of the ruler.

No one will be work with you long term if they don't feel valued by you. They may start with you but drop off the race if they don't feel valuable no matter how much self-esteem they have. Your purpose is meant to help both me and you. If I don't see my use in it I will walk away, not because I have low self- esteem but because sticking with you is betraying me. You are because I am and I am because you are. We need each other's purpose to become all that we can be.

JOURNEY WITH KIKI

She never imagined the first step to volunteer at that organization was going to mark a turning point in her life. Prior to this moment, Kiki had chosen her study program and career based on what she heard would produce swift employment.

She knew she had relatives who looked up to her and her husband for financial support. It never dawned on her to follow her natural instincts and go for who she really is without being swayed by the financial benefit.

The fulfillment that welcomed her in this venture caused her to open a whole new page in her life; one she had shut for so long though the desire had always been burning within her.

REFLECTION

1. What would you do if you silence the voices of your abusers and choose to live for something?
2. Why are you waiting? Are you are expecting something or are you waiting because you don't know which way to go?
3. At this point, what direction can you say your life is heading?
4. Are you living to serve or to live?
5. What are you doing/can you do to fulfill the reason for your existence?

CHAPTER 10:
GOING BEYOND

"Life is a mirror and will reflect back to the thinker what he thinks into it."
—*Ernest Holmes*

Now you have found it, what next? What I can tell you is keep going, no matter what! It is one thing to know your purpose but entirely another thing to expand on it. Your life is about becoming more of who you are, so lengthen your borders.

Most of us, who have lived traumatic experiences, faced devastating situations and encountered violent mind-draining circumstances are waking from what seemed to have been us floating through life yet we do not know how far we can go.

We tend to lack the hope to even think we can ever pursue anything in our life. Some of us, irrespective of our age, achievement and available resources, feel like our lives have been wasted so we just want to settle where we are.

It is time to dream again

Some of us had dreams but through those discouraging circumstances, we have lost our dreams. It is time to dream again. Others have spent so much time pleasing people they have lost what their lives are about. It is time to regain your own dreams for your life.

Do not let your story keep you from your glory!

Do not let your story keep you from your glory! Use it for encouragement, motivation and to push you to rise higher on the ladder of your purpose. Your future is waiting so do not accept any limitations.

Don't settle at the bottom of your purpose. What lies did the voices tell you? They may have said you will never get any good breaks in life so the day you got that job, you said to yourself, "Well this is as good as it could get." Because of that, you settled for the entry level position and never thought you could go higher.

Don't settle for merely telling your story of defeat, victimization, and pain. I respect your story but there is more to your life than that. I want you to raise your head and discover a better life for you.

VISION VS REVISION

While in secondary school and with some courses at the university, whenever we had an upcoming test the instructor used the lessons before the test to do a review of the information which has been passed across. This was done to refresh the students' minds about the past. It may have been a good practice for a specific test but it will not be so helpful if the same material is revisited throughout the academic year.

Do not revisit the unfavourable incidents in your past throughout your lifetime. Live by the dictates of a vision and not the dictates of a revision. A vision is a visit (living) to your future while revision is a visit (living) to your past.

What are the things you keep revisiting? Are they leading you to what you desire or the things you dread? I have come to believe that a person with a vision can stand out in a crowd of visionless people.

DREAM VS VISION

I have used the words dream and vision, which I thought for the longest time meant the same thing, but I later realized that there is a difference between a dream and a vision.

Dreams are things that just come to us as an abstract. It is something intangible we get when an incident or a piece of art ignites a part of us to come alive. Vision is what gives tangibility to that dream. It transforms that abstract into a specific manifestation. A vision is when you add passion to your dream.

Often, we don't have to put in an effort to have a dream. We sometimes dream by default without intentionality. With a vision, we must be intentional; we have to construct what we have visualized. We may not have a picture of our vision at the onset, which makes it is more concrete than a dream. It therefore means that our vision could start as a dream but it moves beyond the level of fantasies by building on those fantasies to produce an image.

A dream ignites in you the things you want to do but the vision reveals the nature of what you can do. For example, I may have dreams of becoming a football player, I fancy running in the field with a ball and other players while a crowd cheers us on. This is a dream but my vision will reveal to me the realities of who I am and what I can do. If that dream is not in line with my abilities, it will end up in stillbirth.

SIGHT VS INSIGHT

Most people on earth have sight to see the things in their surroundings. I say this respectfully, not everyone can see the same dimension. Some can see further than others, some can see nearer than others while others can see clearer. It all depends on the state of our eyes. According to Helen Keller, an American author, political activist and lecturer who was blind and deaf, "The only thing worse than being blind is having sight but no vision." While sight is great, insight is more desirable.

The word insight is derived from two words inner and sight. It is what you see from your inner being, that thing you see so clearly, but the people around you cannot see it. Like sight, some people have an insight of the next twenty years of their life while others can only see the next minute or precisely what is happening at that moment. Your eyes, which are your sight, make you see your immediate circumstances but your insight, which is your vision, makes you see your future. Insight is the greatest asset you need as long as you breathe.

I was uncomfortable to use the word vision for a very long period in my life because my religious mind shaped by some teachings I had heard made me believe that it is a very sacred word reserved to be used only when God takes you physically and shows you a vision. So, there I was waiting for the day God would come hold my hand like he took Abraham, and show me a vision of my future.

As true as it sounds, it is a mindset based on very limited knowledge. Though some people have had the remarkable experience of a physical encounter with a revelation of their future, if God really wanted to visit everyone on earth physically and take them by the hand to show a vision of their future, I don't think He would have left the Holy Spirit to live in is and lead us.

BENEFITS OF HAVING A VISION

An exciting Life: When you have a vision, your life becomes exciting. Vision transports you from that state of hopelessness into a position to look up to life with anticipation. Notice I use the word transportation, which implies that it is a process. If you have a vision today, it doesn't automatically mean you will live in a sustained mood of glee if that really exists.

However, if you have a vision, every year you will have a reason to celebrate an achievement in your life no matter how small that achievement may seem to you. When obstacles come along the way, which will always show up while you go after your vision, the big picture ahead of you will make you see beyond the immediate circumstances.

It determines the depth and height of your purpose: It is what carries your purpose beyond what your eyes can see into the future that you desire. In other words, it is the distance between your purpose and your potential.

You might know what you are here to do but unless you know how far you are able to take it, your purpose will remain as a seed waiting for you to nurture and you can't nurture something effectively if you don't know far it can grow.

I heard the story about the Chinese bamboo. Once planted in fertile soil, it is nurtured like any other plant, exposed to sunshine and watered on a daily basis. What makes it different from other plants is that in the first four years of growing the bamboo, there is no visible evidence of growth. The amazing thing is this, in the fifth year of growth the plant grows to approximately eighty feet in a period of about six weeks.

The only reason the owner of the bamboo tree can keep growing it despite no visible evidence in over four years is because he has a vision for the seed he planted and he knows its potential. When the sower had the seed in hand, he knew the purpose of that seed is to produce a plant. He had a vision that the plant will grow eighty feet tall. Though he didn't see this plant in the first, second, third and fourth year, his vision kept him continuing to water and exposing the "plant" to sunshine. Because he held on to his vision, in the fifth year he had the tallest plant he had probably ever grown.

It will be your motivation: It will keep you going when you feel like giving up. The sower could have given up anytime between the first years when he planted the seed to year five when it sprung up if his vision didn't fuel him to keep watering what seems to be a dead seed. We all need a clear vision because just like an impaired physical sight may keep a person stagnant without the help of an aid, as long as our vision is impaired, we may not go anywhere in life.

Vision gets rid of jealousy in your life: That may not mean so much to you but for some of us this information can be life changing. If you grew up like me, in areas where we heard a person was killed by another person or by a group of people who were jealous of the deceased person's achievements, I can't help but wonder if the killers had a vision for their own lives. If they did, they would probably not have taken the life of an innocent person whose crime was going after his vision.

People tend to be jealous of others because they think others have something they can never have. If they become aware that by developing their vision, they could have those things and maybe more perhaps they will never be jealous of those who have it.

Vision brings provision.

Your vision will cause you to get the things you desire. When you have a vision, you will be busy pursuing it and not looking around for what others have achieved.

I love the phrase that "vision brings provision." We often feel we do not have the capacity to do certain things so we don't venture to go after them. In my experience, when my mind stays on something there seems to be a force which attracts that thing closer to me. I once heard Oprah Winfrey say, "Luck is opportunity + Preparation." Put in the context of vision, when we are preparing to achieve that picture in our insight, the opportunity always falls into place to accomplish that vision.

Along with the opportunity comes the distinguishing factor that sets apart the person who has been preparing with a vision in mind from the one who had no vision and is therefore unprepared to accommodate the opportunity. Have a dialogue with yourself to dig out the vision for your future.

As many are the roles we all play in life so are there many visions a person can have. We need to have a universal vision, which envelopes our entire existence, but acknowledge there are sub-visions that branch out the big picture for every area we find ourselves serving.

For instance, as a spouse, you need a vision for your marriage; though there may be other circumstances your vision will largely determine the outcome of the marriage. Your vision will cause you to work on it or take the exit door when things are falling apart.

If you are a spouse and a parent you need to have a vision for your children, you have the responsibility to train them in the way they should go. You should be able to see things about your children beyond what your eyes can see. See your children in a way that the people around you can't see.

This is what makes a parent to keep raising a baby even when the baby is unable to walk, to talk or to use the potty without assistance. The parent has a vision that the baby will grow out of that stage and do those things that seemed impossible just after birth. Though it doesn't end there, the parent will have to deal with the "terrible twos" and "threenagers" and all the various tantrums that comes between the newborn baby and the independent adult.

A friend of mine once said his grandchildren are the reason he is thankful he didn't give up on his children when he felt like they were too much to handle. To my friend, his vision of having and holding his grandchildren someday was his motivation not to give up on his children but it was more than that, it gave him a direction of where he was heading and how he could get there.

Your vision is a window through which you see into your future.

EXPECTATIONS BRING REWARD

Unless there is a what, there will never be a how yet the how scares so many people to the extent that they fail to see a what. Your vision is what you have seen on the inside, the how are the steps you need to take towards attaining it. That is why you must have an expectation.

If you expect nothing, you get nothing. The reality is not that you got nothing because you really did get something; you simply got what you expected which is – nothing.

I heard a preacher say he kept hearing from many of his parishioners that they don't receive answers to their prayers. Being a concerned and caring leader, he decided with the consent of the people, to closely examine their prayer time unannounced. What he noticed during his observation is that they spent most of their prayer time saying, "O God help me … O God, if you help me … Lord I need your help more than ever …"

During his next meeting with the people, he told them they were very lucky because he realized they had their prayers answered but the problem is they didn't realize they had received their answers. Perplexed, they asked him to explain further because they didn't understand how they had answers they didn't know about.

He went on to tell them that they spent their prayer time asking for help without being specific on what they needed help for. They have received help in one way or another but they didn't get the help they wanted because they were not specific when they asked for help.

In other words, when you have a clear vision of what you see in your future it gives you something specific to focus on and paints a clearer picture of what you expect to get. You won't live hopelessly with the thought that nothing is working for you. On the contrary, you will be excited because as you pursue your vision, you begin to see reasons to celebrate because of the construction of an establishment that initially seemed like a mirage.

TRUSTING YOUR VISION

It is easy to trust your vision when it comes to things like growing a bamboo tree, which some people have grown and can attest that it will spring up after five years. If it easy to trust your vision when the more experienced parents, researchers and books tell you the children will eventually outgrow a stage and hit another developmental milestone, what happens when it comes to the visions that scientifically, medically, and societally seem impossible?

What happens when you see that child who made some poor choices and is currently serving a prison term in corrections becoming a responsible and respectable young man in the next twenty years? What happens when you see yourself running a multi-million dollar business when you currently don't have five dollars to buy a jug of milk and a loaf of bread? What happens when you see yourself alive in the next ten years when the doctors said you only have two months to live? What happens when you are about to commence your dream of going to college but everyone around you thinks you are never going to complete your studies, even the people in authority over you?

Don't judge the possibility of your vision on how other people respond. Consider yourself blessed beyond measure if there are three people who believe in your vision when there is nothing on the outside to show that it is going to be accomplished. The majority of visionaries didn't have the luxury of having two people on their side. I understand that when people believe in you, it gives you the push to press on but when no one believes in you, allow the energy flowing from your determination to come in and push you forward.

Those who don't see a possibility of your vision manifesting to reality may think you are having grandiose thoughts, others will agree with you in your presence but make fun of your vision behind your back while some well-meaning people will try to stop you in the name of looking out for your best interests and the interests of those around you. You will have to believe in your vision for it to come to pass because it will be tested.

I faced a test in the first year of my marriage, when I was pregnant and just moved to another country to do a graduate program. Everything and almost everyone around me told me I could not complete the graduate program including some people in authority with "good intentions". The odds were all against me. I felt like giving up yet when I lifted my head and saw the vision of a certificate of completion that kept me going. It could have been better if that was the only obstacle I had to face.

They had valid evidence to back their opinions while I, on the other hand, underestimated the odds against me. Coming from a society where it takes the whole community to raise a child, I underestimated the odds of raising a child, which turned out to be three children during my entire studies. Faced with a new reality, I only had faith and with that came the provision of strength, resources, courage, determination, and the great support and encouragement of my husband, family from distant lands and good friends I met and made in my new home. This was much more than I needed to accomplish the vision of completing the academic program.

THE GREAT CURRENCY

> The fact that you have a vision is an indication that you have an iota of faith.

Faith is that thrust into your vision. If you want to see your vision come to pass you must be willing to live by faith. You may not know this but the fact that you have a vision is an indication that you have an iota of faith. The reason I am sure of that is because you did not see your vision with your physical eyes, you saw it with your eyes of faith.

That is why you can see what others cannot see and my favourite book in the whole world says if you have faith as little as a mustard seed, you can move mountains. There are so many mountains between where you are now and the realization of your vision so you need to have faith just as much as you need your vision.

Don't walk around saying I don't have faith or that faith thing doesn't work for me. That is a lie your obstacles are trying to make you believe. If you believe it doesn't work for you, it is an indication that you are putting your faith in the wrong place. Why not do yourself a favour by refocusing your attention and start putting your faith in the divine truth, which is the fact that your faith will bring down every mountain between you and your vision.

Now you know you have a bit of faith, you will need to expand that faith to get what you want. I like to look at faith as the currency I use to pay for the things I see in my vision. Everyone doesn't have the same insight to get the things they want because not everyone has the same level of faith.

This explains why two men are working in the same position as entry level sale clerks in the same company, making the same hourly wage. One person says I don't want a lot, my desire is to get a dollar increase and I am okay with that. The other person says I see myself becoming the manager in one of the sales departments.

The difference between these two people is that they have developed their faith to different levels so one can believe for a bit more than what the other person believes for. They both have a vision but their visions are on different levels based on their faith.

If you noticed in the quote earlier, faith is described as a seed. Like every seed, the sower must feed it so it can grow. What you don't feed will eventually die and what you feed will grow, will enlarge, and will expand, depending on the kind of seed you planted. Invest your energy to feed your faith because it is the locomotive to move you to your vision.

When you have a vision, you are hoping for something that is not yet visible. That can be very frustrating, but if you believe you can get it, it takes off the pressure from you and puts it on a force greater than you. Faith is what gives substance to the things you are hoping to get, so go for more of it.

VISION DEVELOPERS

Go Wild and Go deep

The most important feature of your vision is hearing from yourself. We have all been given the gift of imagination. Some people use this and they are called creatives, while others have not tapped into this imagination well so they assume they are not creative. Your imaginative power is your creative ability. We all have the power of imagination so we all have the ability to create.

> Unplug yourself, be still, and connect with your soul to get the direction to your future.

Your vision will not come from your ego, envying others, listening to the opinion of others about your future. It will come through receiving feedback from the eyes of your soul. You can't get a clear message from your imagination if you are busy listening to other voices outside of you. Unplug yourself, be still, and connect with your soul to get the direction to your future. When your vision is clear it will be productive.

You can use your imagination to see want you want. That doesn't mean everything you see in your imagination will be what you get. You will often see things you don't want to see but you can discard that by changing the image or by changing your mind. In other words, you can filter the images in your mind.

When you discard that unpleasant image, use your imagination to create what you want to get. When you get a hold of it, write it down to make it concrete. The more you focus on it the better you get a clearer picture. Napoleon Hill said, "If you don't see great riches in your imagination, you will not see them in your bank account."

UNBOX IT

Allow your imagination to go wild. Get childhood dreams out of the box you have placed them in. I have heard many people say their life is in a cage. Some joke about this, others say it with some seriousness but very few know how to take their lives out of that cage. You may have made such jokes, I put it to you that it is more than a joke, it is a reality.

There is more meaning in the phrase "think outside the box" than the credit we give to it. To have a vision you will have to go beyond the box of your thinking and wander into the world outside the box. The world in which lies the things you think you are not capable of doing. When you come face to face to dreams bigger than your capacity to accomplish, it is an indication that you may have a vision. If your dream is something you can create with your available resources then you are just dreaming and not having a vision.

PASTE IT

You may have also heard that out of sight is out of mind, that may not be true for some things but it is true when it comes to the development of your vision. You can have your vision in your mind's sight always by affirming your vision, writing it down or if you are a visual person like me get a vision board. Practice whatever appeals to you in order to paste your vision in your mind.

Affirming your vision doesn't mean you go out there looking for anyone who cares to listen so you can tell them your vision. You affirm your vision in private. Make it a daily practice, choose a specific time and place when you will read your vision to yourself. The more you read it out the clearer it becomes and the greater the chances of it being real.

Also, when you write something down, it sinks in deeper. However, it is not enough to just write down your vision, you must write down the reasons why you want to achieve it. Your reasons will motivate you when the odds start rolling in. There will be voices that will say you don't deserve to have what you are going after, voices that will cause you to doubt yourself and wonder if you are on the right path. That is the moment when you pick up the reasons for your vision and remind yourself why you need to accomplish that vision.

So, if you want to do something you have never done before to get something you have never had, search within yourself for a powerful why. So many visions have gone down the drain because the visionaries did not have a strong why so they dropped along the race, therefore giving the obstacles an upper hand over them. You are too great to let the challenges let you down.

There is an anonymous saying that "When life gives you a hundred reasons to cry, show it that you have a thousand reasons to smile." You may not be able to count to a thousand reasons but there is a big reason, which could not be measured up with a thousand reasons. Find it and keep it before your eyes.

An image speaks millions of words. In my elementary language lesson classes, the teacher used to give us a picture to describe in our own words. All the students received the same picture but every student composed an essay based on their interpretation of that image at that time. Each time you look at the portrait of your vision, not only does it give you the complete picture of what you are pursuing, it also allows you to dream of several ways to get it. When I face an obstacle while am going after a vision, I usually pick up a picture of what I want to get. While focusing on that picture, ideas start roaming through my mind. At that time, I can pin down one or more of those ideas to resume the journey to my destination.

Plant yourself in the environment that causes you to dream big. It is in our nature to hang around people who make us feel good and make us feel we have great accomplishments. That is awesome, we all could use a boost of cheers when we attain success, but if you want to go higher than your current circumstances, hang around people who challenge you to dream bigger than your current situation.

Sachin Tendulker, a former cricketer and captain, credits his success to his brother and coach who made him push higher by not appreciating his last success. Sachin said, "If I score runs, let the rest of the world talk about it. I think about the next game … We don't talk about the last game, we talk about the next game."

Your environment goes beyond the people you meet in person periodically. In this digital age, it goes into your social media space and your web environment. Steve Maraboli said, "If you surround yourself with clowns, don't be surprise when your life resembles a circus." Look for experts in the areas of your interest, listen to them daily, read their books and learn from them for you will become like the people in your circle.

Stay close to people who uplift your passion to accomplish your vision and those who will give you constructive criticism. Criticism will always come and you don't have to listen to them but you need to have people whose criticism you keep and not just toss into the garbage. Filter the criticism in the same way you filter your imagination.

JOURNEY WITH KIKI

The product of decision is one amazing mystery, one that spins a life around to an unfathomable destination. Despite the challenges in her life, Kiki's passion for helping others lured her to act on her unquenchable desire by applying to graduate school to become a therapist.

Her ability to see that she could do much more with her life spurred her with a push of hope. It seemed like the gates that kept her bound to her past in her present had suddenly flown open catapulting her to a future she had never thought possible.

What seemed like her current limitations became so blurred to the extent that all she could see was the despair of others being broken.

REFLECTION

1. What are some deep questions you can ask yourself?
2. What are your strongest desires?
3. How do your fears limit your expansion?
4. Are there any risks you can take towards your future if you know for sure that you are not going to fail?
5. What is the area of your focus? How does it bring positive energy into your life?

CHAPTER 11:
THE JOURNEY CONTINUES

I'm sitting down by the seashore on a beautiful cool evening, absorbing the fresh air blowing across me by the generous wind while my hands feel the sharpness of the sand and my eyes simultaneously wandering around with admiration of the magnificent trees swaying to the direction of the breeze. The refreshing breathtaking environment seemed to have got a grip on me until I was brought back to the awareness of my surroundings seconds later or perhaps minutes later when I realized I had ben staring intensely at the faraway land miles across from my sitting position.

Back to reality, my interest drifted from the beauty around me to wondering what could be on the other side of the ocean. I wanted to see the mountains that were glancing over the water. The thought of going on a first hike caused a smile to escape my lips along with an urgent rush of excitement flooding my heart. I wanted to see the city whose inhabitants were staring at the same ocean like me. What kind of city would it be? Was it mostly populated with tourists like my habitat or did it have more locals who enjoyed the hunting trips in the heart of the mountains?

As I allowed myself to travel with the waves into the world way beyond my physical eyes I said to myself, the other side of the ocean doesn't have to be my stopping point. I could discover a greater part of the world by taking a longer trip than a few hours drive to the mountains. It will be a rewarding adventure to go places; it would be life-changing to meet another slice of the world. Unsure of the full reward of the trip, one thing is certain: adventure never comes alone. It always brings a host of lessons, some we use to move forward others we ignore and remain in the same spot waiting for a better opportunity to utilize them or maybe we just discard them for forever.

Now within me lies the burning desire to go on an adventure. How do I get there? Contacting a cruise agency to go far away to distant lands could be a good start. Taking a long road trip along the borders of the sea and visit the neighboring mountains I first dreamed of could be another option. Irrespective of what I choose, my bag of lessons on the side of the world will have to begin with a choice. I could choose to sit on that bank all day imagining what may or may not be, but to experience it I need to get started.

Life is a journey. On this journey are three groups of people. Group A knows where they are going and how to get there. Group B knows where they are going but do not know how to get there. Group C does not know where they are going neither do they know how to get there. These three groups of people have certain things in common: intentionality, planning, programming, and commitment. Some have discovered them and are practicing them, others have discovered them but are still to use them while the third group is still to discover and take advantage of them to get to the destination the way they want to get there.

INTENTIONALITY

The logic is that we are all on a journey, and we will arrive at a destination irrespective of if you choose your destination or not. Those who choose intentionally will be satisfied with the outcome at the end of their journey while those who are passive will wish the outcome was different, or like we sometimes put it: we will wish we could turn back the hands of time. Now is the time to turn your wishes into satisfaction by being a person of intentionality. When we fail to choose intentionally we are left with no choice but to accept everything that comes our way then blame the outcome on time and chance.

In John Maxwell's words, "Wishing for things to change wouldn't make them change. Hoping for improvements wouldn't bring them. Dreaming wouldn't provide all the answers I needed. Vision wouldn't be enough to bring transformation to me or others. Only by managing my thinking and shifting my thoughts from desire to deeds would I be able to bring about positive change. I needed to go from wanting to doing."

> I had the power to turn the tables around and become a lead character in my story.

In unintentional living, life happens more to you than you happen in your life. In other words, you are a spectator in your own story. That was the story of my life for as long I can remember the greater part of my life. I would wait for time and chance to heal my wounds, I would wait for opportunities to come to me, I was basically a participant while waiting for everything else and everyone connected to me in one way or another to run the major aspects of my life. If you have ever had a glimpse of such a life, you will attest to how frustrating this is, yet, unknown to me I had the power to turn the tables around and become a lead character in my story.

I would imagine myself being free from the dictates of my circumstances but I couldn't imagine myself moving on to create that freedom. The torment of living under that bondage weighed me down more than the events that had caused me to lose my ability to take control over my life. Deep within me, I knew I could become more than who I was but I lacked intentionality because I thought I was in a safe spot so moving out of it could be taking myself into a danger zone.

My thoughts were can I trust my ability to make decisions? It could be a lot better to let others run my life than trying to take control of my life and fail. I feared defeat more than attempted success though George Edward Woodbury says, "Defeat is not the worst failures. Not to have tried is true failure." I saw some truth in those words so after battling with myself for so many years I finally took the great step towards intentionality.

PLANNING

That step was to make a choice to have my own vision and stick to accomplishing it. As a person of faith, I always knew God has a plan for my life but I failed to understand that he doesn't plan the plan for me. That is where so many of us miss the mark. We failed to see the difference between God's plan and us bringing that plan to align with my life. I thought if He has a plan then it will come to pass somehow, I don't have to play a role to make my life better, it will get better with time. Boy, was I wrong! My situation went from bad to worse because the anxiety of waiting for desires to be fulfilled caused negative emotions to mount up and have an upper hand over my best reasoning.

The vision you have for your life could be small in your eyes or too big for you to believe it will happen, but the fact that you choose to have a vision is a big step, which must be applauded. That notwithstanding, no matter how exciting the vision for your life is, frustration will set in if you don't have a plan on how to accomplish it.

As a teenager, I used to think planning was meant for the government officials who design the city and give their consent for buildings and roads to be constructed. The only knowledge I had of planning then came from the town planning office in my city, where individuals registered their lands and obtained approval for construction. Living at that time with my grandmother who was a farmer, I could not miss this information because she always went to the town planning office whenever she purchased a new piece of farmland.

Now I sigh at the limited knowledge I had on planning. Knowledge is the key that determines the height of life by the depth that is acquired. Shallow knowledge will produce a low life. We often use low and high to explain our state but rarely do we realize that it is associated with our estate.

> You can take control of your own life through knowledge.

A person is in a high state when they have consumed more quantities of a substance, in the same way, a person can have a high estate by consuming more knowledge. The more you know the more achievements you call into your possession. Value and maximize the opportunities to gain knowledge not just waiting for time and chance to bring in your desires. You can take control of your own life through knowledge.

As good as knowledge is, it also has its limitations. According to Jim Rohn, "Don't let your learning lead to knowledge. Let your learning lead to action." That is where planning sets in. To move from the stage of merely learning to the stage of implementing knowledge, you need a plan.

A person may have an intriguing vision in the area of his purpose but both the purpose and vision will head towards a natural death without a plan. A plan therefore speaks life into purpose and vision.

Benefits of planning

The years I spent living with my grandmother shaped my life in more ways than I can imagine. As I observed her life as a farmer and trader, I learned some lessons, which didn't seem to mean a lot to me at that time, but applying them to my life later is yielding more fruit than I would have thought.

My grandmother never had any formal education in a classroom or online on farming and business but her success as a farmer and trader was remarkable because she lived a well-planned life. Some of us struggle to plan our day or week but my grandmother didn't only have her day and week planned, she also planned her year before she started it.

She knew the crops to plant in the different months of the year and had mastered the crops that flourish in the various seasons. In some months of the year, she would plant the seasonal fruits and vegetables, harvest and sell them when they are in demand. As the season closes, she doesn't sit and wait for the next season to plant that same product, she obtains the seeds of the next seasonal goods, plants, harvests and sells when they are in demand. This circle goes on all year by rotating the fruits, herbs, spices, and vegetables.

She even went the extra mile to know the products that flourish in her city of residence and those that produce better in the soil of the neighbouring cities. As it is, where there is excess the value reduces so the purchase price is lower and where supply is lower demand is higher. My grandmother who has never seen the four walls of a classroom or owned a computer in her life is the smartest economist I have ever known. She would carry her excess products to sell in neighbouring cities where there is more demand at a higher price. On her way back home, she buys the products that are excess in supply in that city to sell in her home city where there is more demand and makes profits in the process.

Planning brings excellence in any area of your endeavours. You do not need a plan if you want to live a mediocre life, neither do you need one if you want to live from hand to mouth or grow your own food and be the lone consumer. You do need a plan if you want to stand out in the crowd.

My grandmother lived in the urban city. It is a city of thousands of people so it is unlikely to be popular in the city unless you are a politician, footballer, musician or someone of outstanding achievement. However, my grandmother is one of those people whom you don't need to know her address to find her house. Not because she lives in a castle but because her trading excellence made her standout in the city. She was popularly known by the name given by her customers "Mami Douala," than her real name.

Douala is the city where she would buy the products that flourished in its soil, to resell in her city of Buea. As such, those who couldn't travel to Douala to buy for themselves anxiously waited for her return to have what they need. **They could trust her timely delivery** because she didn't just travel to Douala randomly. While planning her week, there were days scheduled to work on her farm, days to sell in Buea and days to travel to Douala. Her customers knew the days they could meet with her to get freshly transported goods. ***Thus planning always leads to consistency***.

Planning brings growth, which is easy to miss because some of us have the mindset that growth brings planning. We are accustomed to laying back and say when our businesses, careers, or family grows to a certain level, we will plan on how to manage it. That is a vision heading towards failure. ***A plan sets the foundation*** for something to grow out of. You probably have heard a business owner say, "I built this business" or a parent say, "I am building my family." They are both right. Your vision will not spring out of nowhere; it takes building upon each step of a plan to come up with a fully constructed life or business. I chose to look at a plan as a block because we must put each one in its place to see a beautiful structure.

It helps you have a focus for every area of your life be it in career, family, marriage, or business. A few months ago, I was having one of those mother-daughter conversations with my mother. One thing she said that made me realize how far I have come in my recovery journey is that she mentioned she was going through her phone text messages and email. She was marvelled at the many different careers and jobs I told her I want to get into. She said every month it seemed I came up with something new, which I was certain was THE thing I want to do.

At that point in my life, I had been intentionally taking control of my life. I wanted to be more than just living; I wanted a different outcome than the direction I saw it going. However, I had no plan on how to get to the broad vision I had so everything that came into my mind and what was proposed to me seemed to be the perfect way for me to get to the vision. The day I finally had a plan on how to get to my vision everything changed for me.

It seemed a test was being thrown at me as almost all the people whose opinion matters to me had great ideas for me to implement and get to my vision though some of them had no idea of what I had seen for my life. Their ideas seemed great but most of it was out of my plan. This doesn't mean a plan cannot be altered. It means any alteration you make should tie with what you want for yourself for as they say, "You are the master of your own destiny." Now I am focused so I can examine the ideas from well-intentioned people.

It guides you to maximize your resources and eliminate waste. Have you ever felt like time flies, money gets in your hand and falls out under your palm, perhaps there is a hole in your pocket or leakage in your bank account? Opportunities come in, which could take you to the next level but they pass by unutilized. I have been there far too many times than I can count with the fingers on my hands and toes put together.

To get to the destination you see, you must be a great steward; one who manages time and resources to have a great return from your input. A great plan involves estimates on time, money and other resources. In this generation flooding with information, there are many resources to help with time and money management. Talk to a trusted person in the area of your interest to get the best resource needed for your recovery.

GET IT IN AND GET IT OUT

The mind is very powerful, not only does it determine our attitude but it gets to set the pace for our life. How fast or slow we go in life is determined largely by how much we are willing to put our mind to work. For most of us, we have had others act on matters that concern us because we didn't feel worthy enough to speak out. When I decided to be the master of my own conclusions, I started by listening to the advice of people who always had the final say in my affairs. I listened, pondered over it and took action centred on my values.

However, I do admit that some of us are struggling with unhealthy thinking. It doesn't come easy for us to just accept advice, ponder over it and act. What comes naturally for us is to focus more on the negatives because through no fault of ours, those traumatic events distorted our thoughts and beliefs. However, we must challenge our thinking so we can get out of that trap of struggling to the place of our dreams.

When it comes to writing our plans, we may think "Good things never come our way" so we drop the paper and pen because we don't see why we should spend our precious time to write something that may never happen. When those thoughts come in, we must challenge them because according to Cognitive Behavioural Therapy that thought is a product of overgeneralization.

You may have valid reasons to think defeat and failure are supported by evidence of something that happened in the past. It costs us so much to invest our interest in achieving a goal so it is normal to be devastated when the interest is not rewarded with accomplishment. The truth is you may have failed at something but that doesn't make you a failure. I am sure if you retrace your steps, you will see instances of success along your path.

For the sake of rising from the position you are in now, do not disqualify the victorious moments in your life. Dwell on and build on them as a motivating factor for you to write out your plan as you see yourself having a similar or greater victory in the future.

Therefore, to come up with your action plan, you must think. Think about the things that matter most to you. The career you would like to have, the kind of family you want to build, what you consider your safe zone, safe environment and decide what a fulfilled life means to you. This was very challenging for me because the traumatic incidents in the first decade of my life swallowed my healthy thinking ability so I lived more by instant and impromptu actions.

You can jumpstart the thinking process by asking yourself personal questions like, "Who am I?" and "Where am I going?" Ponder over these questions and write down the answers that flow into your mind. Think about where you want to be in the next six months, one, two, five or ten years from now. Whatever you write down doesn't have to be a finished product. Be open to refine it in the days, months and years ahead as the vision becomes clearer or twists with occurrences.

When you choose to write your plan, keep in mind that there is no perfect environment to write down your plan, different places work for different people. It is easy to get stuck in this initial stage of choosing the right environment so always remember this to minimize feeling overwhelmed. I normally like a quiet room away from distractions and responsibilities. Others like to sit in the woods or close to a lake. Do whatever is needed to sharpen your mind for the ideas to flow in and for you to identify them.

> **To identify your unique plans, you must be true to yourself.**

To identify your unique plans, you must be true to yourself. This is not a time to think about what your family and friends think about you; what society did wrong to you and how people react towards you. It is a time to think about what you want for yourself and how to get there. It is a time to know how to do the things that inspire you. There may be many routes to get to your vision but not all the routes are rewarding, neither are they all in line with your values. Seek clarity on knowing what route to take.

If at this point in your life, you cannot answer the question of what you see your future looking like, it is an indication that you are not the person at the centre of your life. You have handed the power to events, circumstances, time, chance, and other people. As such, it is time to have a personal plan for your life.

BE INVOLVED IN GOAL SETTING

Plans are programmed by breaking them into goals. Goals are the steps necessary to fulfil your vision. You can have a plan for the next five years of your life but your goal will tell you what you do today to get aligned with your plan in fulfilling your vision. After writing your plans, start with a goal of glancing at it daily. The more you look at it the greater the chances to reach or refine it.

Goals give the specificities of your plan. For most trauma survivors, the best place to start in moving forward to the vision of our life is to have a wellness goal. I used to think wellness means losing weight and eating healthy but I have come to realize that wellness is the vital choices we make towards becoming a better version of ourselves. It encompasses issues like how we recognize and respond to our emotions, and practice self-care.

In my case, one of the things I didn't consider as part of wellness is a sleep pattern yet that is something most of us struggle with. When it was time to sleep, I would have a recap of all the things that have gone wrong in my life that day and link them to the events of the previous years. Before I know it, I have starved my sleep to death. Since I am fully awake, I turn to television and movies as a better option to keep my mind busy, giving me something to feed my mind as opposed to the thoughts of defeat and failure. That may not be a bad idea except that the movie keeps me awake to about 3:00 a.m. and I had to be up by 6:00 a.m. to start the day.

I understand that people have different sleep patterns based on reactions to medications and other factors. This sleep pattern is an example from my personal struggle which was purely affected by toxic thinking. It is by no means any suggestion to recovery but a guide.

An important item on the plan for my life was to have a better sleep, which was very vague until I set a goal to go to bed at 10:00 p.m. and wake up at 6:00 a.m. To accomplish this goal, I had to find something that relaxes my mind and gets it ready to rest. We all have different relaxation techniques. My go-to activity to relax my mind is the meditation on scriptures. Having that specific time goal and relaxation activity made my plan prolific.

That was my starting point but over the years I have had to refine the goal to fit into circumstances like being pregnant, having children, waking up and going back to sleep at their schedule. At this point in my lif,e I go to bed way earlier and wake refreshed. However, the initial goal of a fixed bedtime and relaxation technique placed me in a healthy sleep routine.

Breaking our plans into goals sets us to succeed with the plan. Another plan I also had was to have a healthy weight and have more energy. When it came down to breaking the plan down to goals, I had to determine where I was at and where I needed to be to have more energy. Without that, I could lose one pound, which means my plan is accomplished but I still won't have more energy so it will not be realistic to say I had succeeded at my plan.

On the other side of it, we do not want to set our goals up for failure and get our mind into the spiteful reinforcing cycle of being incapable of accomplishments. Let the goal be something you can do and not something you dream of doing. For me, I dream of spending one hour in the gym six days a week but it will be unfair to myself if I set that as a goal because I can't keep up to that at the current stage of my life and fitness level. Yet, if I fail at it, I have set myself to receive the blame for not being capable to meet up with the task. A better goal would be to set a time frame to walk few minutes a day then build on that foundation.

One of the most important aspects to achieving goals is to have a motivating factor for that goal. If you want to move on with your life after that difficult situation, have a strong why for wanting a better life. When you face challenges; which will always come, pick up your written reasons and read it to inspire you on the journey.

Inspiration also dwells in a community that shares your goals. Besides the community being an inspiration for you to accomplish your goals, it will also provide you with valuable resources and support to overcome your challenges.

On the way to getting the big reward of having your vision accomplished, reward yourself for every accomplishment. We are often hard on ourselves for the mistakes we make. It will be so much better if we can check for the gain in the mistake and reward ourselves for it. You deserve it so go for it!

JOURNEY WITH KIKI

When Kiki first had her target to volunteer, it was challenging to her. Although she once had the burning desire to work, events of the last few years plunged her to the state of not wanting to get out of her house. She had to force herself to go out on some days because she had to take her children to school on the days she didn't cancel their attendance.

She knew what she wanted but how was she going to act on it? Her first goal was to take her children to school on every school day if both she and the kids are healthy. Keeping up with this goal motivated her to add an activity to do while her children were at school; this is where she fits in her volunteer activities.

Inspired to leave the house daily, she began to set other goals to achieve a good personal hygiene. Also, the joy generated from her service motivated her to do more. This gave birth to her vision of becoming a therapist.

It is amazing what planning, the accomplishment of what we consider a tiny goal can birth. She noticed that as she began working on herself by setting goals to meet the needs of her spirit, soul and body; everything else in her life started falling into the place she desired but thought impossible.

Today, five years after her initial contact with the lady, she is a licensed therapist and friend shining her light on others. She Loves. She Lights. She Lives!

REFLECTION

1. Has someone ever asked you what your plans are for the weekend? Well, today I put it to you: what are your plans for your life?
2. Do you have any experience with goal setting? What are your good and bad news about it?
3. How does a life of intentionality sound to you?
4. What end do you see from your beginning?
5. How can you get there?

EPILOGUE:
LIVE YOUR LIFE

Life can be challenging but you don't have to face it alone. Like Bobbi Parish, founder of The International Association of Trauma Recovery Coaching and Trauma Recovery University always say, "You matter, I am here, I see you, I hear you, and I care." Those are not just words; there is truth in every one of those words. Somewhere around you lives someone who genuinely sees you and your value.

Don't let the history drain the energy for your destiny. You can dream again, get the life you desire and deserve. I pray that the knowledge you have obtained from this book will not only be for information but for implementation.

However, if you have any form of hesitation to implement, then there is still one thing you need to conquer: fear! Irrespective of the reason you may have for not taking action, fear is the underlying factor. What is your greatest fear?

- Do you fear to dare out of familiarity?
- Do you fear criticism?
- Do you fear to let go of your past for an unknown future?
- Do you fear failure?
- Do you fear success?

You have to confront your fears if you want to release your giant. You are not the ant trauma made you believe you are. In every giant, there is an ant but you have to find your lost GI to reinstate yourself to the giant you were.

Your GI is your greater intelligence. It is the intelligence that does not come from the books you have read or the opinions of other people. It comes from your inner being. It is the intelligence that flows from who you are within, the weightless person you are when everything else vanishes.

Among the millions of people who will read this book, each word will have a different meaning to each person. This is because every individual's greater intelligence will speak to them differently based on their aptitudes.

Add your GI to the ant you think you are and you will see the giant that has been caged for too long come to life in the area of your interest: your career, business, family, health, and any area of your life.

Do not die an ant! Test your limit to see how far your potential can go. You have the greater intelligence to be much more than you can ever imagine. Your imagination is only a starting point.

Do not stand at the bars of your dream, staring at the place you want to be. They hurt you once, maybe repeatedly but do not let them hurt you forever. Break the emotional cage. Go! Find out what is beyond that barrier. Go and thrive.

ENDNOTES

1   Douglas College. *What Is Psychosocial Rehabilitation?* Retrieved from https://psyrehab.ca/pages/what-is-psr (PSR/RPS Canada, 2013). Accessed August 21, 2018.

2   Skye Barbic, "Personal Recovery Outcome Measure (PROM)." https://www.psyrehab.ca/files/documents/ENGLISH%20 VERSION.pdf Accessed November 12, 2016

3   Susanne Babbel, "The Connections Between Emotional Stress, Trauma, and Physical Pain." *Psychology Today* (Blog, April 8, 2010). www.psychologytoday.com/ca/blog/somatic-psychol-ogy/201004/the-connections-between-emotional-stress-trauma-and-physical-pain Accessed August 21, 2018.

4   Brene Brown, "Living Brave with Brene Brown and Oprah Winfrey," (published on Nov 23, 2015). https://www.youtube.com/watch?v=oidZ-XESijg. Accessed November 3, 2017.

5   https://www.merriam-webster.com/dictionary/paradigm%20shift

6   Aaron Orendorff, "The 7 Best Lessons From the 7 Best Business Books of 2017 (So Far)." *Success* (Blog, June 12, 2017). https://www.success.com/the-7-best-lessons-from-the-7-best-business-books-of-2017-so-far/ Accessed on June 13, 2017.

7   Holly Burkhalter, "It's the 21st century. Yet slavery is alive and well." *The Washington Post* (Blog, June 27, 2017). https://www.washington-post.com/news/democracy-post/wp/2017/06/27/its-the-21st-century-yet-slavery-is-alive-and-well/?noredirect=on&utm_term=.85a47c59b23b Accessed September 05, 2018.

8   Vanessa Van Edwards, "How not to give a damn about what others think of you in order to be fully free?" (Blog, April 26, 2017. https://www.quora.com/How-not-to-give-a-damn-about-what-others-think-of-you-in-order-to-be-fully-free Accessed April 30, 2018.

BIBLIOGRAPHY

Oprah, Winfrey. (2017). The wisdom of Sundays : life-changing insights from Super Soul conversations. NY : Flatiron Books.

Patrick .,W. Corrigan; et al. (2009). *Principles and practice of psychiatric rehabilitation : an empirical approach*. New York : Guilford Press.

ACKNOWLEDGMENT

With special thanks:

- To my Creator for planting this book in my heart. You brought me back on track when I tried to run away from the task. You led me through the entire process. Truly with you nothing is impossible.
- To everyone who shared their stories, struggles and success of trauma with me. You are amazing! Keep shinning your light.
- To my husband, Samuel, for your unwavering support, love and leadership.
- To my children Felicia, Manuella, Joshua and Elizabeth; for helping with the realization of how to love so I can serve well.
- To my mother, Eyong Helen Besem, for your unconditional love and for believing. You set the right foundation for me.
- To my British Columbia Psychosocial Rehabilitation Advanced Practice family, especially Dr. Regina Casey and Jenn Cusick, your support exemplified a true PSR strength-focused approach.
- To a talented and outstanding publishing team, Ari Miller; FriesenPress publishing expert, Mary Metcalfe; FriesenPress editor, and Alyssa Doucet, FriesenPress Designer. Your consistently positive input, good eye, sharp mind, emails, calls, patience and creativity led to the development and delivery of this work.

CPSIA information can be obtained
at www.ICGtesting.com
Printed in the USA
LVHW030143190319
611082LV00001B/44